Advances in Human Understanding
Stories for Exploring the Self

John G. Watkins, Ph.D.

Crown House Publishing
www.crownhouse.co.uk

First published in the UK by

Crown House Publishing Limited
Crown Buildings
Bancyfelin
Carmarthen
Wales
SA33 5ND
UK

www.crownhouse.co.uk

© John G. Watkins 2001

The right of John G. Watkins to be identified as the
author of this work has been asserted by him in accordance with
the Copyright, Designs and Patents Act 1988.

All rights reserved. Except as permitted under current
legislation no part of this work may be photocopied, stored in a retrieval
system, published, performed in public, adapted, broadcast, transmitted,
recorded or reproduced in any form or by any means,
without the prior permission of the copyright owners.
Enquiries should be addressed to
Crown House Publishing Limited.

British Library Cataloguing-in-Publication Data
A catalogue entry for this book is available
from the British Library.

ISBN 1899836756

Printed and bound in the UK by
The Cromwell Press
Trowbridge
Wiltshire

In Memoriam

TO FIG
Who shared with me
His dreams.

I never had a brother
And always wished for same
In garb of new-found friend
One day my brother came.

Adventures left our cares behind
We searched for secrets of the mind
Together gleaned what we could find
Discoveries shared for all mankind.

Closeness marked our passing years
Today's no time for fear and tears
Who knows perhaps 'twill simply be
Adventures new for one to see.

Table of Contents

Preface by Woltemade Hartman, Ph.D. iii
Acknowledgments v
Introduction: Startin' Time vii

Part I: The Springtime of Life 1

Chapter 1 The Flagpole 3

Chapter 2 "Cool" 13

Chapter 3 The Ballad of Billy Brown 19

Chapter 4 Unconscious Communication 35

Chapter 5 The Nerd 41

Part II: The Summer of Life 75

Chapter 6 The "Hero" and his "Sister" 77

Chapter 7 The Novel 85

Chapter 8 The Therapist 103

Chapter 9 The Cuckoo Bird's Egg 121

Part III: The Autumn of Life 147

Chapter 10 Andrew and his Old Sheepdog 149

Chapter 11 Buddies 155

Chapter 12 Dao-Tsai and the White Marble Image 173

Chapter 13 Quittin' Time 191

Chapter 14 The Clock 195

Part IV: **The Promise of Life** 217

Chapter 15 **The Golden Journey** by Jack D. Watkins 219

Preface

"Leave a trail of wisdom …"

A small telescope once brought visions of celestial worlds to a young boy … and the desire for "wisdom" impelled this boy's later move to academic halls. However, he soon discovered that universities teach only knowledge, not wisdom. As a young man of serious mind, like a true Dao-Tsai, he searched for "The Way"—what man's striving is all about. He traversed "The Way" for many years and discovered that all life is a promise, a challenge, an exciting exploration, and that one must become a complete individual on one's own in order to experience true oneness with a universal ocean of life energy. This man is John G. Watkins.

To write a preface to this book is indeed a great pleasure and an immense honor. John Watkins had become a mentor, guru, father, artist, teacher, friend, trainer and colleague for many, and particularly for me. Many have been inspired by John Watkins's therapeutic self, his resonance and humanity in helping people to recognize the multiplicity of their inner resources and to actualize their potential. One realizes while reading this book that the author had a much greater purpose in mind than adding just another book to his impressive list of academic and scientific contributions.

Adventures in Human Understanding is a book written in the spirit of humanism. It is a book about life, about being human, and it cultivates not only a reawakening of what we are—our self, but also an understanding of fundamental human values such as faith, trust, hope and above all, the interdependence of humans on each other. It is written in a time when love seems to be fading and hatred and despair rising, when human values are forgotten and only differences remain. The stories told in this book rekindle a sense of values and a respect for the dignity of humankind. In a way this book is a contribution to *Wirklichkeitsanalyse* as it explores and analyses the psychosocial factors involved in human existence. The author describes life as a golden journey, a discovery of self-energy, resources and potentialities implicit to each human being. The book is surely a helpful guide as one continues upon the journey of being human. I hope and trust that this book will have a formative influence on all those who read it.

Finally, the book reminds one of an inevitable "quittin' time." However, *Adventures in Human Understanding* will leave a trail of wisdom for future generations ... that "life should not merely be valued for its quantity measured in chronological time, but for its quality measured in experiential time."

Woltemade Hartman, Ph.D.

Acknowledgments

The author will be forever indebted to the people who shared with him the various sides of their personality and events in their lives. Some of these events were true, some partially true, and others completely fictional. They were aspects of life, however, which go to make up human existence.

These "events" were occasionally observed (and sometimes participated in) by the writer himself. Often they were told to him by high school, college and graduate students plus associates, friends and colleagues.

Patients in psychotherapy represented another source. Some of these were soldiers in the army, inmates of installations in the Veterans Administration, clinics, hospitals, prisons or drawn from private practice. To protect their privacy I have commonly changed names and places.

Above all, I am enormously indebted to Helen, my wife, sweetheart, colleague and "in-house" editor. At times in the past she has been my co-author. Not only did she add, subtract, correct and assist in fashioning this work but, as an experienced psychologist and psychotherapist herself, she contributed sensitive, clinical insight in depicting various "cases," and their psychological understanding.

Introduction: Startin' Time

All life is an exploration, right from the start. Some folks believe this beginning occurs when a sperm and an egg cell embrace. Others think it's when we leave the warmth of our mother's womb. Either way, it's "Startin' Time," and the adventures begin. When the cold, cruel air of the delivery room first hits, some of us make loud protest with a cry and vigorous kicking. Everybody is then pleased, and the little bundle of joy begins its life journey by exploring the world, with lips, fingers and feet.

Each adventure brings a new and expanding universe, such as crawling away from mother's watchful gaze or climbing out of the playpen. It's all exciting and largely filled with fun. The more we learn, and the broader our world, the bigger as persons we become.

Many years ago, a very small boy in a very small town had a very big present given him by a very caring father, a teacher. It was the gift of learning how to read—even before he went to school. Fresh vistas were opened. Not only could he grow by personal experiences, but he could also enjoy events lived-through by others.

In a compulsive ecstasy this lad visited the town library, established by a Mr. Carnegie, who had acquired a fortune and was now giving it back before he left for parts unknown.

Each volume in this small collection revealed a new adventure. How exciting! It fired frequent visits (almost one every day). Once kindled, a burning thirst for "knowledge" can never be quenched.

A small telescope brought visions of celestial worlds, and a desire for "wisdom" impelled the boy's later move to academic halls. However, universities teach knowledge, not wisdom. The facts of knowledge are like jigsaw-puzzle bits, pieces that must be connected into meaningful patterns to achieve understanding. Like rain from heaven, wisdom comes not by choice nor by conscious effort, but it may drench us as a by-product of exposure.

Adventures in Human Understanding

As a youth, whose altering physiology diverted attention from outer worlds to inner ones, the science of psychology offered to this young man a new challenge. He wanted to discover what goes on in that little black box, the brain, that determines how humans behave.

Later, as a young teacher, he shared the fears and hopes of hundreds of high school and college students. Finally, as a mental health professional, he combined academic research with listening to many "patients" in hospitals and clinics, who might reveal the secrets of their lives. What they told him constitutes the building blocks for constructing the various stories here inscribed.

Violent and exciting episodes in which the hero foils international villains are popular today. But none of the people who inhabit these tales is a patriotic superman battling evil conspiracies, attempting to overthrow the government, provoke nuclear destruction or enslave the human race. These pages are filled with the experiences of normal people, who doubt, fear, love, hate, strive, triumph or fail in their quest for happiness and meaning. Some of them pursue unrealistic, immature goals. They grasp for money to satisfy excessive greed, or seek to acquire power regardless of consequences to themselves or others. At times, destruction and death result. And some fail because of unjust treatment through no fault of their own. There is no attempt here to make justice prevail simply to please our sense of rightness. Life is not always fair. But the aim throughout this work is to stress a sense of values, one that upholds the essential dignity of mankind.

Not all of the tales have happy endings. Some of our storybook characters acquire wisdom. They pursue lives of contribution and meaning to themselves and others. Perhaps the greatest achievement by some is to understand "love" and the ability to give and receive it with friends, family or life partners. Occasionally, their "friends" are not even human, but nurturing others, called pets.

Our "heroes" range from the exuberance of youth, through the trials of mid-life crises, to those in the autumn of their existence, squeezing the last drop of juice from the fruit of life before winter arrives.

Introduction

The "Startin' time" for some described herein was near the turn of the nineteenth century; for others, it was during the mid-decades of the twentieth century, and for some it was more recent still. One, "Dao-Tsai," centuries ago searched for meaning in his existence—as today we still seek. "Human Nature," while ever evolving, also remains much the same. The children of yesteryear encountered hope, pain, rejection, striving, success, failure and the proving of self-worth much as we do today. Their experiences are still relevant.

A few of the stories depict real-life experiences of the characters. Some tales are partly true and partly fictional, while others are the product of imagination which have been constructed about the lives of people who impacted the writer as associates, friends, students and patients. In these cases, events may have been altered or names and circumstances changed to protect their privacy. But the abiding criterion for inclusion is that each should in some way offer an "adventure in human understanding," one to which a reader might relate.

The stories are interspersed with brief essays and poems that amplify our search for human understanding. Finally, since many of the life problems here depicted involve unconscious as well as conscious motivations, brief "Thoughts of a Therapist" have been added. These analyses-and-comments sections aim to provide rationales as a therapist or psychoanalyst might evaluate the characters and their situations.

When "Quittin' Time" finally comes, perhaps we can see it as only leaving one global playpen for a fresh and larger challenge, an exciting new exploration. Among all those who have gone before, none has come back, so we do not know what is there. We may hope and wish for a paradise filled with pleasure or to avoid a nether region of pain. But maybe our existence simply merges into a universal ocean of life energy—a view that many would protest. At least we know that each of us must first return to our own "Startin' Time," the bosom of Mother Earth. But why should this be filled with fears and tears? It just might be the beginning of an exciting new adventure.

Part I

The Springtime of Life

Chapter 1

The Flagpole

"Betcha I can." "Betcha can't." "Betcha I can." Two teenage boys, wearing the green "beanie" caps that identified their lowly status as new students at the College, were standing beside the flagpole arguing. Eldridge, in a moment of bravado, had just informed his buddy, Herman, that he could climb that gleaming metal pole. It was six inches thick at the base and reached as high as the three-story Administration Building behind it.

Rolling green grass blanketed the campus, framing the three primary buildings of the college, conservatively constructed of brick. This 400-student college was respected as a center of culture and education in the agricultural valley. Isolated from large metropolitan centers, its faculty and student body formed close relationships. People knew each other.

Sporting large rimmed glasses, red-faced Herman was short, stocky and auburn-haired, while Eldridge, tow-headed and more angular, was the string-bean type. Both wore suede jackets and tan corduroy pants typical of the day.

They strolled toward the "men's" dorm. Herman was not about to let Eldridge off the hook.

"You're so smart, El. You think you can climb that pole. I dare you to."

Eldridge, caught unexpectedly, wasn't sure he could really climb that formidable tower of steel. But now it had reached the point of "a dare." There was no backing out without losing face. Like that time in the third grade when Harley had put a chip on his shoulder in the schoolyard and dared Eldridge to knock it off. Even though Harvey was bigger, El had swung his arms faster, and had bloodied Harvey's nose. The shouting boys quieted down, and all

Adventures in Human Understanding

agreed that El had won. He had learnt that you mustn't be a coward and back down. Besides, it sure felt good when you won.

But now self-doubts arose. El wished he had kept his mouth shut. The more he looked up at the flagpole, the higher it grew. When you're in a weak position, you attack. So, shifting ground, Eldridge raised the ante.

"Maybe we could make it like a contest with the sophomores."

"What do you mean?" queried Herman.

"Well, suppose we get some kind of a flag, a freshman flag, and tie it to the top of the pole," suggested Eldridge, trying to enlist Herman as a co-conspirator. If the project failed, Herman would be at least partly to blame. El explored this new idea further.

"We could dare them to get it down. Wow! Supposing they couldn't do it?" Eldridge, sensing Herman's interest, continued his sales pitch.

"Those sophomores, especially 'Con' Shore (their class president), think they're so smart and important. Do 'em good to get sat on their ass."

Herman nodded agreement. Now the stakes were really high. Eldridge could end up a hero to the whole class, or a bum who had failed. He absolutely had to climb that pole.

Mildred, a tall freshman girl with long dark hair rippling over her shoulders, had been following them and listening to their conversations. Suddenly, with great excitement, she broke in.

"That's a great idea. I can sew up a green flag with 'Freshman Class' in white letters. You can tie it to the top of the pole, El, and we'll really put down those sophomores." Now the battle for prestige was really joined.

Eldridge was sweet on Mildred and had planned to ask her out for a Coke-date at the Pie Lady's, who sold candy and soft drinks in a remodeled home just three blocks off campus. If he failed to climb the pole, he would not only lose face in front of Herman and the rest of the freshman class, but also before Mildred. There would be no Coke-date.

The three partners in crime conferred on the details of their enterprise and agreed to keep it secret as to who was involved. However, Eldridge had already made up his mind. If it was successful, he would leak the identity of the "hero."

It was 4 a.m. on a frosty November morning. Ding! ding! ding! went Eldridge's alarm clock. He struggled to reach over and turn it off. Every fiber of his body was numb. Maybe this whole deal wasn't such a good idea. Then he thought about his commitment to Herman and Mildred, the time she had spent sewing the flag and what it would mean to his standing on the campus. Wakefulness dawned slowly. Finally he stretched alert.

Donning an old pair of blue Levi's and a raggedy shirt, he threw over his shoulder a faded bag, which said "Saturday Evening Post" on one side. It had sat idle in a dresser drawer for several years, ever since Eldridge had surrendered his "Post route" to a younger boy. Vacillating between excitement and worry that he might fail, he set off for the campus several blocks away.

The temperature was well below freezing. There was no snow, but heavy white frost covered fences, trees and parked cars. Not a soul in sight as he approached the flagpole.

Before starting to climb, Eldridge checked the contents of his shoulder bag: Mildred's green flag, a piece of baling wire, a pair of white canvas gloves, a small glass jar into which he had poured some thick, dark molasses, an open can of axle grease and a typed notice, which read, "The Freshman Class were men enough to put this flag on the pole. Let's see if the sophomores are men enough to get it down?" El gleefully visualized their discomfort. "Wow! They sure will be pissed-off."

He started to squeeze the little tube of glue, brought to attach the notice to the pole. In a second thought, he decided he'd better not stick it there until he had really finished the climb and attached the flag. Maybe, just maybe? But he mustn't forget to glue the message on the pole before he left.

Next, he put on the white canvas gloves. After pouring molasses on them, and also on the knees of his Levi's, he started to climb.

The going was more difficult than he had planned. He would hitch his knees up, reach higher with his gloved hands, grasp the pole a few inches above, then pull himself to a higher level. Foot by foot the ascent progressed. The cotton gloves did not keep his hands warm. They felt like blocks of ice.

Darkness was beginning to fade. A slight glow appeared in the eastern sky, just enough for him to read his wrist watch. Almost five o'clock. He'd better hurry. Although it was early somebody might show up on the campus. Even Dr. Salomon, the English professor, who usually came to his office before any of the students, shouldn't be arriving yet.

Reassured, and with increased vigor, he resumed climbing. The last two feet were agonizing. Ah! the top of the pole. Reaching in his shoulder bag, he pulled out Mildred's flag.

With his knees tightly clamped, and holding onto the ice-cold metal pole with one hand, he desperately tried to fasten the flag to the top of the pole.

"Why wouldn't that piece of coat-hanger wire bend? Damn! There! Got it."

He dipped a gloved hand into the can of axle grease.

"Look out! Almost dropped it."

Finally, scooping up a glob, he slowly slid down the pole, spreading the grease with both hands.

"Boy! Am I tired. It's late. Get going or someone will see me."

As El started home he thought, "Just time for a good snooze before that nine o'clock math class."

He had gone only a few yards when he suddenly stopped. "Oh yes! Almost forgot to glue the note on the pole."

Rushing back, he squeezed the tube and stuck the message some five feet from the bottom. In ten minutes he was home and in bed. The covers were hardly pulled up when, reveling in the glow of success, he succumbed to the urgings of Morpheus.

The sun was shining in El's bedroom window when he startled awake. Half-dozing, he thought, "Oh-oh! That nine o'clock class. What time is it? Ten thirty? So what?"

He jumped out of bed. Having accomplished very important things, it was time to find out the result.

At the campus, a small group of students were milling about the flagpole. A few chuckles from the freshmen. A few snorts of disgust from sophomores. Who the devil had put up that flag and that notice? Soon the speculation turned from "who" to "how." How could anybody get the flag down? It was obvious the greased pole was unclimbable.

But the honor of the sophomore class was at stake. The flag had to come down. Moreover, that green flag up there should not be permitted next to the American flag, which was raised each morning. It was a matter of national patriotism. Furthermore, lowly freshmen could not be permitted to gloat over their superiors. New ideas and reinforcements were needed. A conference of Con Shore and other sophomore leaders was held.

Joe, a husky upper classman and tackle on the football team, suddenly came up with a brilliant idea.

"Listen guys. Why not let the I-Club handle this matter?" A growing number of sophomores were suddenly all ears.

The I-Club was composed of men who had received school "letters" for athletic participation. It was governed by the most prestigious players, the "jocks" and the campus "heroes." The I-Club maintained campus "discipline" and ruled with an iron hand. Severe punishment was meted out to any freshman boy

Adventures in Human Understanding

caught on the campus who was not wearing his green "beanie." During noon break the offender was forced to lower his pants in front of the Administration Building. A severe paddling was then administered by members of the Club. After one such experience, very few of the freshman boys forgot their beanies.

The I-Club thought Joe's suggestion was a great idea. Insurrection at the lower student levels could not be tolerated. The freshmen had created the problem; let the freshmen solve it. An announcement was made in assembly and reinforced by a notice on the campus bulletin board that read: "Unless the green flag on the flagpole is removed within 24 hours, every freshman male student will be paddled in front of Sterry Hall."

Like the flowers in spring, smiles blossomed on sophomores throughout the campus. The freshmen would get what they deserved.

Among freshmen, consternation reigned. Either they, the freshmen, got that flag down or they faced severe corporal punishment. Eldridge was especially disturbed. Now he was in a pickle. Instead of being a campus hero, he would be blamed for all the trouble and for the paddling his classmates would receive.

Another conference of war was held. Freshmen leaders, including the girls, tossed about ideas.

"Just leave it there. We can't let the sophomores win."

One skinny little boy replied, "Yeah! but you girls won't get paddled. We will."

Somebody shouted, "Who put it there? He oughta take it down."

Another grouched, "The smart-ass who dreamed up this trick is responsible."

But almost everybody agreed, "The sophomores couldn't have done it. They're cowards for calling the I-Club."

The Flagpole

Mildred was one of the leaders among the girls who argued this way.

After no solution seemed to be found, Eldridge spoke up.

"It's not our fault we have this problem. But we've got to get the flag down. How about asking the City Fire Department to come to the campus, put up one of their tall ladders, and remove it." With cheers and noddings, this idea was acclaimed by all.

The City Fire Department was approached. After hearing of the situation, the firemen were amused. As a group devoting their lives to rescuing the helpless, they sympathized with the underdog freshmen. Their biggest truck came to Campus Circle the next day, the ladder was raised, and the flag pulled down—to the cheers of all onlookers. No charge was made to the College or the freshman class.

The campus returned to its normal routine. Classes were held on time; class rivalries resumed, and the I-Club members continued to win glory for the school. Herman, Mildred and Eldridge mutually agreed to keep the secret and never reveal who had put up the green flag.

One evening, a year and a half later, they were celebrating Eldridge's admission to the college elite. Mildred looked admiringly at El's new purple sweater with the large yellow-gold "I" on it.

"It sure looks good on you."

Eldridge smiled. He had been a successful wrestler in the 125-pound class.

Sitting at the only table in the small room, Eldridge turned toward the owner and ordered, "Coke, please." The Pie Lady dutifully reached in the cooler, extracted a bottle, pried off the cap and handed it over with two straws. Eldridge bounced a quarter off the counter. Mildred, now increasingly knowledgeable in what pleased the male ego, added a deft touch.

Adventures in Human Understanding

"You sure pinned that guy from Whitman College. It took only two minutes."

"Yup. He thought he had me when he got a full Nelson. Didn't know how strong I was."

Eldridge smiled broadly and flexed his biceps. "Maybe climbing that flagpole helped build my muscles."

The conversation turned to the depression. Eldridge opened. "It's getting real tough. My uncle had to sell his potatoes at fifty cents a hundred-pound sack. Some of his neighbors said they weren't worth picking these days. Told anybody who wanted to come and help themselves. If the bank hadn't renewed the mortgage he'd have lost the ranch."

Mildred's tale of woe was equally sad. "My Dad's a carpenter. Nobody's building houses these days. He's out of work half the time. If it doesn't get better, I can't go to school next year. I hear the tuition will be fifty dollars higher."

"Don't worry," put in Eldridge bravely. "President Hoover will stop the depression soon."

Mildred felt a bit argumentative. "Maybe we need some new ideas—like what that guy Roosevelt is talking about?"

Eldridge scowled. Girls didn't know anything about politics. "Roosevelt's a radical socialist. You can't fiddle with the economy. We've been studying the law of supply and demand in Econ. class. Hoover's got the patience to sit it out. You wait and see."

Mildred liked his confidence, even if some of his opinions were rigid. She changed the subject. "I see the I-Club paddled three freshmen at noon today."

"Yup. Those kids were getting too smart for their own good. One of them thought, because he weighs 220 pounds and is slated to be on the first team next year, he didn't have to wear his beanie. We showed him how wrong he was."

Mildred didn't respond at once. Two more sucks on the straw. Finally she looked at him with a mischievous smile. "You didn't feel that way last year. How come you changed?"

"Well, now that I'm a sophomore I've grown up. I see matters in a different light. Didn't realize then how important campus discipline is."

Mildred could barely muster a "hm."

The straws were now making sucking sounds, but yielding no Coke. They walked back toward the campus. On arriving at the girls' dorm, Eldridge planted a luscious kiss on Mildred's lips. It could have gone on longer. But Mildred, hearing the sound of footsteps, suddenly realized it was ten o'clock.

"The Dean of Women. She's going to lock the door. I gotta go." Breaking off, she dashed inside just in time.

Eldridge made his way slowly toward home, musing to himself. Now, having arrived at a position of respect, status and power, not to mention wisdom, life had few problems—even when you had no money.

Thoughts of a Therapist: Analysis and Comment

The problems faced by teenagers today are similar in many respects to those confronting adolescents a generation ago. The needs to establish independence from adults and to prove masculinity in boys have been ever present. The early rites of courtship and mating were less direct then but still progressed through recognized stages. Overt sex was infrequent, but bragging was a commonplace activity.

Athletic prowess then, as now, was highly prized, and those who excelled were held in high regard by classmates. Competition was keen, and less gifted students had difficulty establishing status. In our hero, Eldridge, we see all these motivations operating.

Now, with high-speed cars, easily available guns and drugs, adolescence is a much more dangerous stage than ever. "Dares" today can result in challenges to "face," which are taken out in gun battles, not mere fist fights.

Bragging sometimes led to over-commitment. Failure left one lower on the totem pole. While he doesn't want to completely humiliate his friend, Herman's small stature ensures that he will probably not attain the desired status of an admired athlete. With Eldridge's over-commitment, Herman is in the one-up position and wants to make the most of it. Eldridge skillfully displaces the issue to a higher plane—which appeals to Herman.

Once Mildred enters the picture the problem becomes one of do-or-die for Eldridge. In adolescents with less-sturdy egos, failure in such a situation might eventually lead to suicide—as it does in later stories. Still, even now the game is for real, and the stakes are high.

Eldridge plans well and, with a super-human effort approaching the limit of his endurance, he succeeds in climbing the pole. The result, however, is unexpected to the three conspirators. Eldridge, who has everything to lose, comes up with a good solution.

One and a half years later, Eldridge, demonstrating the flexibility of youth, identifies with the I-Club athletes and reverses his beliefs (re: "campus discipline"). He is apparently unaware of his inconsistency, which is apparent to Mildred. She enjoys teasing him—one of the few ways girls had in those days of expressing aggression. When she confronts him, he rationalizes his change of belief by claiming greater maturity—which is not apparent.

A simple problem and a simple solution leave Eldridge feeling smug. For a while he will not need to brag. The reinforcement of success makes him stronger to cope with adversity as an adult. His over-confidence, however, may lead to a future downfall. He meets potential failure realistically and overcomes adversity now. But how will he hold up if faced with a real failure in the future?

Chapter 2
"Cool"

A young teenager Henry was
A freshman in the school.
He looked at all the boys around
Like them he would be "cool."

The captain of the football team
The leader of his class
The guys at whom the girls made eyes
With status that would last.

He learned the most important thing,
'Twas seldom taught in school.
You'd never ever count for much
Unless they thought you "cool."

Now Mother said your homework do
Come in at ten each night
"Uncool" that was and often did
Provoke a family fight.

At thirteen he had dragged
A cigarette, Kool Light.
And now at least a pack a day
To him seemed almost right.

Grandpa, a man he dearly loved,
Had smoked for many a year.
But told him it was bad for you
So what? He had no fear.

Old codgers wouldn't know what's "cool"
You need not pay them mind.
The guys all puffed at each school break
He'd not be left behind.

Adventures in Human Understanding

Last year he had a sobering jolt
When Grandpa gasped for breath
And said, "I've often tried to quit."
'Twas a month before his death.

Then, one bright day the guys smoked pot.
It was against the rule.
But Henry never passed it by
'Cause that would not be "cool."

And when there was a football game
They'd drink the cheapest beer.
You only had to lie your age
At a grocery quite near.

One night he got so sick and drunk
He hardly got to school.
He did his best, but flunked the test,
'Cause an "A" grade wasn't "cool."

But when he took the driver's test
He followed every rule.
And so got passed as one of the best
For the right to drive was "cool."

Then one fall night the gang was tight.
Got stoned with crack cocaine
All five of them, while Henry drove.
Devoid of any pain,

Would shout and yell at the passers-by
Insulting words. 'Twas fun.
Until another gang gave chase
And after them did run.

Of course they didn't wear seat belts
Though scolded by their Ma
For only sissies wore such belts
Although it was the law.

They sped the highway 90 per
The other gang to fool
So they at school next day could brag,
And show that they were "cool."

The curve was somewhat icy
When Henry jammed the brake
His old car drifted off to the right
The turn it didn't make.

Now Henry knew just what to do,
To slow there was no need.
You spun the wheel to the other side
Without reducing speed.

But somehow when it crossed the line
While weaving back and forth,
It hit head-on with a grinding crash
A Chevy traveling north.

Both of the cars rolled off the road
One person was alive,
The driver of the other car
But no one else survived.

Now Henry and his four young friends
Will go no more to school.
But though they're dead, it could be said
They sure were plenty "cool."

Thoughts of a Therapist: Analysis and Comment

In the poem *Cool* the excesses of modern adolescence are demonstrated at their worst. Instead of the earlier "age of innocence" exemplified by harmless pranks, we now have a tyranny signified by the word "cool."

"Cool" in modern teenage culture means conformity to whatever is defined by this generation as desirable. The same need for independence from parental control is now manifested by submission to peer control. To be "cool" may mean acting different from the teachings of parents and other adults, even to the point of self-destruction.

These rebel behaviors may include smoking, drinking, drug abuse, staying out past suggested curfew, refusal to complete school assignments, academic failure, or racing on highways minus the protection of seat belts, to name just a few.

The teenager's drive for independence and need for peer acceptance is normal. It is a way to find out who he or she is as a separate individual from the parents. It is the road to adulthood that every teen needs to take to reach maturity. Who am I? What are my values? What do I believe in? What are my goals? In what way am I different from the adults in my life?

As each teen struggles with the same questions, whether conscious or not, they are drawn together in their own value system, currently called "cool." This is a normal process only if the past guidance of parents and teachers is not automatically discarded and the new culture of "cool" overwhelmingly adopted. Such a teen remains a child because his past dependency is simply replaced by a new one.

But why would a teen become so rebellious? Apparently his past experiences have not given him a feeling of inner strength, a feeling of confidence, a feeling of acceptance. So he seeks teen-acceptance with other teens, and the culture huddles together to seek reassurance from each other.

Most parents do the best they can in raising their children and are often puzzled by their teenagers' behavior. Every human being lives within his or her world of perception, and it is not easy to understand how a child may see things. For example, a father may work long hours for the benefit of his family, but a child may feel neglected and uncared about. As a result, the child will feel unworthy, unimportant, unloved. Even with the best of communication (though very important), perceptions often go awry.

When the striving to be "cool" becomes a tyrant, it may carry a young person to destruction as it did to Henry and his four friends.

Chapter 3

The Ballad of Billy Brown

I
This tale's about a football game
And a lad of great renown.
It's oft retold in somber frame,
The Ballad of Billy Brown.
Young Billy, brightest in his school,
A genius for his age.
In science he outstanding was
And always made "A" grades.
Of Galileo, he would dream
Plus Jupiter and Mars
Or Einstein, who made sense of things
Uncovered in the stars.
And Billy always won the prize
At the county's science fair
Where every one competed by
A gadget made with care.
Some said he'd get a scholarship
And surely wouldn't fail.
Perhaps at noted Harvard,
Columbia or Yale.
It would have been a happy end
To the saga in this tale.
In form our Bill was very slight.
He also looked too pale.
That lacking in much strength or might,
He'd probably avoid a fight,
'Cause he was very frail.
Ignored by others in the school,
And thought by all a fool.
So when in a class,
Choice of partners was cast
He always was passed,
Until at the last

Adventures in Human Understanding

The only one left in the pool.
And rarely a girl,
Gave him time or a whirl
When weekend parties arrive.
For seldom he dared
And was never prepared
A heart-breaking "No" to survive.
He'd rarely walk with other boys
And his voice was seldom heard
Awkward with a lack of poise.
And so they called him "nerd."
A sensitive heart young Billy had,
So when his thoughts got really bad
He'd dream of the day, when coming his way
His exile would end, by finding a friend.
Then his night would be turned into day.
Of course there was Lottie,
Who never was haughty,
And sometimes spoke in the hall.
"Hi Bill," she would say,
When he passed her each day.
And once on a hunch
She even ate lunch,
And then let him carry her tray.
His heart was a-flutter,
But all he could utter
('twas only a mutter)
Just "Hi," and pass by
For nothing more he could say.
Then this gorgeous beauty,
Though really not snooty,
Gave a smile as her duty
And tripped down the hall
On her way.

II
Now Valleydale High,
Sitting top of the hill,
Could its destiny fill
Without people like Bill.
While far down below,

The Ballad of Billy Brown

Forever its foe,
The common folk's school,
Whose students weren't "cool,"
Surrounded by shacks,
Where the people drove hacks,
And worked with their backs
Lay the Riverton School.
One day when his team
Practiced football it seemed
To Bill walking home
By the field
That each student's kick
Looked like it was sick,
Went far to the side
With too short a glide
And rarely made more
Than an infrequent score,
Which the coach would ignore
And seldom a point did it yield,
Completely missing,
Or just barely kissing
The uprights at end of the field.
Then Bill blurted out,
With almost a shout
And startled the folks
That were standing about
"I'll bet I can kick it
And much better stick it
Between those posts on the line.
Then it will go straight,
And never be late
In clearing the bar every time."
Bill felt very scared
And aghast that he dared.
When silence preferred,
As he shouted this word
Hostile feelings bestirred
Much wrath from the herd
For which he'd never prepared.
"Ha! What a dumb nerd,"
Said Charlie McCurd, the quarterback he

Adventures in Human Understanding

While many who heard
Passed down his sharp word
And the rest simply chortled with glee.
"Get out of our way,
We've got football to play,
And too much to do,
To waste time hearing you,
Blocking kicks is our job
For today."
But one of the coaches
Stopped all their reproaches
And playing his hunches said
"Let's let the kid go.
And put on his show,
It might get some sense
In his head.
Put the ball down
On the thirty-yard line.
Now Billy just wait
'Til I give you the sign.
The center will pass you
The ball from behind.
Then you will soon find
That it baffles the mind
To kick and score points
Every time."
The ball it was passed,
Which he instantly kicked
With all of his might and main.
The orb soared high
Way up in the sky
'Tween the goal posts so far
It sailed o'er the bar.
And three points that team
Would obtain.
When tackles dived at him
Intending to flat him
Bill feinted a step to the side
And the movement confusing
Which caught them both snoozing
Brought a laugh

The Ballad of Billy Brown

That the coach couldn't hide.
Through all afternoon
Bill kicked more, and soon
The balls flew fifty yards far.
It looked quite deceiving,
But all were believing
For every one sailed o'er the bar.
The coach was convinced
And told all those near
That Bill their kicker would be
For the rest of this year
And the team gave a cheer.
A shout which filled him with glee.

III
In the school's corridors
And on all of its floors
The girls smiled at Bill passing by.
As he walked down the hall
He no longer felt small
'Cause often they gave him the eye.
Lottie even went with him
A student dance to attend.
And Bill now basking in her smile
Was happy for a little while
Cause he had found a friend.
Throughout the year
He played each game
And built the team's high score
With three-point goals and touchdown points,
But there was even more,
Like when he'd kicked some sixty yards, and then
The ball was seized by Milltown's end
Who ran it through the entire team,
And would have made a score
That could have lost the game for them
But Bill who standing there, just then
Did tackle him, though twice his weight
The whistle blew. The game was through.
And Milltown lost by ten to eight.
Our Bill was carried from the field

Adventures in Human Understanding

On shoulders of a sturdy mate.
And all the town, with joyous sound
A day and night did celebrate.
Once when he to the barber went
To get his hair trimmed short
The barber said to him,
"Of course, football is just a sport.
But you'll get honor in this town.
We hope you stick around."
And then his coach the paper wrote. A column did it fill.
"This kid, our kicker Bill, will bring
Our Senior High much fame.
And if he keeps it up next year,
He'll go to Notre Dame."

IV
Then so the days through autumn passed,
And everywhere was cheer
For soon the Christmas joy approached,
As always now each year.
The shops were filled with happy throngs
Plus wide-eyed girls and boys
And Santa Claus in every store
To them did promise toys.
But three weeks 'fore the Yuletide came,
One hurdle must be tried
Their last and greatest football game.
The champions would decide.
The finest school in all the state
Would Valleydale get the crown
Or could there be the slightest chance
For yonder River town.
Unthinkable the school agreed.
"Our team will put them down."
The County Fair had started there,
With prizes going round.
And the big parade began its trek
On the stadium's parking ground.
While on the first float Bill appeared
Surrounded by the team.
The people cheered when he went by,

The Ballad of Billy Brown

The entire town 'twould seem.
And then when evening came that day
The stands did early fill.
With every seat full occupied
Despite December's chill.
The coach told them that winning
Was not their only aim,
And then he said that "football
Was only just a game,"
But still, he made it very clear
That he expected them to hear
From all the people of the town
A bursting cheer, when a win was near
And Riverton put down.
And finally then he told the team
That they would always win
If they'd hold fast to the goals he'd set,
And which he knew'd be surely met,
And rarely ever should forget
That football strife is the game of life
To win or lose they should decide
And never from their duty hide
Then they would be on victory's side.
And now with championship so nigh
They'd surely never let some shame
Ever enter the game, or sully the name
Of Valleydale Senior High.

V
Now when the team came rushing in
And onto the stadium ground
It was a wondrous sight to see
Folks shouting all around.
With clapping hands to the marching bands
As they strode on the playing ground.
So bright and bold in green and gold
While Valleydale's flag they did unfold
Amidst the screaming sound.
But when the cream of Riverton's team
Came walking on the field
A roar of boos dogged every step

Adventures in Human Understanding

To tell them they must yield.
Then in the air a coin was thrown
And Riverton won the toss.
Came from the crowd an audible moan
At e'en the slightest loss.
But spirits high the game began
'Twas even more restored.
When one of our team
Grabbed a pass that soared
Ran down the field,
And then he scored.
Approval loud the people roared.
Came now a light and grayish mist
The sun, its face with darkness kissed
The field befogged both far and near
Without clear sight Bill's kick was missed
For him the first in all the year.
The coach, however, felt no fear
For there would be more chances clear
And times for scores that could be got.
So worry now would be for naught.
Then back and forth the game it waged.
No score for either side.
The script it seemed as if 'twere staged.
Like changing of a tide.
Three quarters passed, when at the last
Five minutes still remained
Then Riverton a fumble grabbed
And length of field it raced.
The score for them was seven now
With a kick that was well placed
Then Charlie McCurd long passes made
And the team ran the ball to the four.
Though try as they might with the goal in sight
They could not move it more.
So Bill was called, two seconds left
To kick as his final chore.
And when he ran out, the crowd gave a shout
That grew to an ear-splitting roar.
For who could doubt, that this was about
The championship and more.

The Ballad of Billy Brown

Then just as Bill was set to kick
Time out did Riverton call
With hope that he would nervous get
And let them block the ball.
So on the sidelines then he paced
With lectures from the coach
Who said he could redeem himself.
It sounded like reproach.
Then someone from the crowd came near
And passed to him a note
In Lottie's hand he clearly saw
The message that she wrote.
"You'll kick the goal, if you love me,
And champions our school will be."
He crumpled it in shaking hand
And dropped it on the ground
Then with his foot he stomped it down
While he was looking all around
To see if someone standing near
Saw down his cheek, there coursed a tear.
He brushed it slowly with his hand
Then strode out where he'd make his stand
And confident he did appear.
A silent calm went all around
With a thousand breaths on hold
And when the ball was then put down
(As later it was told)
Bill kicked it high up in the sky
A winning score foretold.
When suddenly a Western breeze
Rushed in as if a giant sneezed.
The soaring ball was seen to freeze
As the gust of wind its orbit seized
And threw it down on the crossing bar
While a thumping sound heard near and far
Informed that it had bounced again
And everyone knew who heard that sound
The winning score did now depend
On where the ball would finally end.
In front or just behind
Where the goal posts stood

Adventures in Human Understanding

That really it should, and surely it would
If everyone there would focus his mind
And force that ball to fall behind.
Then o'er the crowd swept a horrible moan
Which one can't really describe
While thousands let forth with a ghastly groan
Which made Bill feel he was alone.
Swept up in a raging tide.
Gloom and despair spread all around.
While tears from many streamed down
For dreaded most, in front of the posts
The ball lay dead on the ground.
Then Bill unbelieving
Thought his eyes were deceiving
As heaven crashed down from afar
His head seemed on fire
As he sensed the team's ire
'Cause the ball never crossed o'er the bar.
On the other side of the stadium field
The Riverton team showed the power they could wield
They jumped up and down, then paraded the ground.
And pulled down a pole at the goal.
With sarcastic taunt their prowess to vaunt,
They waved on high the champion's cup,
The trophy they had just stole.
Then Bill humbly ambled off to the side,
And slumped on the bench where his team would reside
Though many strolled by, not a soul lingered nigh
His mates merely stared, while the coach really glared
And Bill found no place he could hide.
For now he felt shame at losing the game,
That sullied the name of Valleydale Senior High.

VI
Then later when he reached his home
His mother looked away.
From her he heard no kindly word
For nothing she did say.
But his Dad looked sad,
Though not real mad, and said:
"Guess you did poorly today.

The Ballad of Billy Brown

So what? You can wait.
Sometimes it's just fate.
But never too late
To prove you are great
And do it in some other way."
Discouraged and weary Bill went to his bed
And never woke up 'til the morn.
But when he arose, and put on his clothes
He felt like his soul had been torn.
He must go to school, and try to act cool
So his friends there would know what a terrible blow
To his hopes and his feelings of shame.
'Cause he'd tried his best, just as much as the rest
At yesterday's football game.
Pondering fate, for his class he was late
The first time he'd broken the rule.
He slunk in his seat, so none he would meet,
That morning in Valleydale School.
Ignored by teachers and all of his mates
And especially by friends on the team
Their eyes seemed filled with dagger-like hates
He wished somehow he could scream.
Gone now was his fame, for he'd brought shame,
To Valleydale High and sullied its name.
There was that one, but only one
Who kindness gave to him
'Twas she who taught his science class
A lady tall and prim.
"Hi Bill," she smiled and softly said,
"Some day you'll know when this is past
That football's only just a game.
Respect yourself. You weren't to blame."
But later in the day he met
Fair Lottie in the hall.
She looked at him straight in his eye,
Then slowly turned and passed him by
With never a word at all.
At two p.m. he felt so crushed
He strolled away from school
And sat alone in the city park
Just feeling like a fool.

Adventures in Human Understanding

And finally when the shadows came
He slowly walked toward home
Not knowing really what to do
Or whither he could roam.
The door he opened very slow
And saw no one was there
Which seemed to him another blow
His pain alone to bear.
A note he saw upon the table
"We've gone to Grandma Brown's
Because, you know, she's hardly able
To Christmas shop in town.
We'll stay the night and play some bridge.
You'll find there's chicken in the fridge."
And it was signed, "Love, Mom."
Then finally when darkness fell
He had to go to bed.
But restless dreams and horrid schemes
Kept running through his head.
He saw himself back on the field
To kick the winning goal
A thousand times he did it o'er
But it was not for real
'Cause every time cruel waking came
The score from him would steal.
Down from the hill the Christmas lights
Were sparkling o'er the town
While drinking cheer, both far and near
The carolers went round.
They sang of peace, good will to men
And then he heard a bell
No ease from it he found
It seemed to toll like a funeral knell.
A slow and somber sound.
But finally just before the dawn
When darkness still was holding on
He woke and felt his thoughts were clear
That he must somehow end this year
Down to his parents' room he went
Asearching through their closets bent
'Till what he sought, just like he thought

The Ballad of Billy Brown

There in a box and laid in a drawer
Was hid his father's forty-four.
It would be used to shoot
A burglar in the head
Whoever tried to rob their house.
At least that's what his father said.
Then Billy slowly climbed the stair
And went back to his room
With key in lock most carefully sprung
He spoke a prayer that he had learnt
When he was very young.
The phrases all he did recall
Came quickly to his tongue.
He then knelt down beside the bed
With clasping hands he finally said:
"And now I lay me down to sleep
I pray The Lord my soul to keep
And if I die before I wake,
I pray The Lord my soul to take."
Then just before the rising sun
He lay down on the feather bed
And put the pistol to his head
The gun went off with a deafening roar
As his blood so red, gushed out from his head,
While his brains spilled over the floor.
The boy we knew had crossed the bar
But maybe from his place afar
Great Galileo watched and heard
The lonely cry of a dying "nerd."
And had him carried to that star
Where cutting words can never scar.

VII
The next day when his folks returned
And tried the bedroom door
His father went and got the key
And wondered "What's the score?"
But when they opened up the door
To see what they would find
His mother fell upon the floor
And shrieking lost her mind.

Adventures in Human Understanding

Bill's father slumped in deepest gloom
His sobs completely filled the room
Grim sadness ruled them night and day.
'Twas said it never passed away.
The folks in town were horrified
At what young Bill had done.
Was this because the championship
Their team had never won?
And most asked why when they passed by
The school and felt the shame.
Could it really be that all this pain
Was caused by just a football game?
But when they went to bury him
There were but few who came.
And as the village barber worked
Upon an oldster's head
He'd tell the story of the game
"Dumb kid," he often said.
Fair Lottie grieved perhaps a year
But never seemed to smile.
And then she married the quarterback
To live in handsome style.

VIII
Football, you know, is just a game,
And fame won't pass you by
As long as you will cause no shame
Or never ever sully the name
Of Valleydale Senior High.
And that's the tale that's often told
Throughout the entire town
Of a football game and a fragile lad
Who failed his team when his kick went bad,
And couldn't live it down
By many folks who think it's sad
The Ballad of Billy Brown.

Thoughts of a Therapist: Analysis and Comment

Billy already enjoys youthful success with recognition that he will probably graduate from a distinguished university and take his place in society as a respected scientist.

However, during a boastful moment his previously unrecognized athletic ability in a restricted but highly valued skill is discovered by the football coach. He becomes almost overnight a community "hero."

The motivations of his school and community capture his entire attention. His normal need for peer approval receives popular acclaim by his ability to "score points" through kicking a football. This community praise reflects the aggressive-competitive society of the country, where professional athletes are paid millions of dollars when they win, but cast aside when they no longer win.

Billy is drawn into this social milieu and for a time enjoys his "hero" status. Classmates and the community praise him. Attractive girls seek his company.

It is precisely because he has reached the pinnacles of school and community adulation that his fall from that peak, through no fault of his own, becomes so devastating.

The acceptance of his world shows its hypocrisy. Because he fails to kick the winning score in a single "championship" game, he is rejected by almost everyone, the coach, the team, his classmates and the community. The platitudes so mouthed, that "winning isn't everything," are revealed as false. Winning is everything.

His athletic prowess has replaced his previous scholarly successes. It has become his world—which is now destroyed. At this point he is in most need of support, and it is almost entirely lacking. He is rejected by all, and most painfully by his girlfriend. One teacher offers support, but it alone is insufficient.

His well-meaning and loving parents are absent at precisely the moment he needs them. They recognized his disappointment, but they did not listen enough to comprehend his total despair. They evaluated the magnitude of his disappointment by realistic adult standards, not those of a vulnerable teenager.

Depressed youths often signal their need through prior suicidal gestures, but people do not hear the "pleas for help," before it is too late.

Suicidal depressions often occur when everybody else is most happy. At Christmas the stricken individual becomes aware of the contrast between his or her own misery and everyone else's joy. Death is very attractive then. When nobody else loves them, "God will receive them."

Billy's suicide devastates his parents. They will never fully recover. The community feels some guilt as it senses its false overemphasis on winning. However, it takes no real responsibility. To lose has brought "shame" to "Valleydale Senior High." He pays the penalty. People forget and go on with their lives.

Chapter 4

Unconscious Communication

We humans like to think of ourselves as logical beings, knowing ourselves and understanding a world which was created for our convenience and enjoyment. When science challenges any of these beliefs, we resist. Mankind has suffered three great insults from scientific findings that were not in accord with long-held convictions.

A great fury was raised in religious circles when Copernicus first published a book concluding that the earth was not the center of the universe, that it and all the other planets revolved around the sun. Galileo, an astronomer with a telescope, made observations tending to confirm this position. He was forced to apologize and repent such views by the Inquisition on pain of being excommunicated as a heretic.

The second insult occurred when Darwin published findings indicating that we were not special beings, created in seven days by God, and in His image. We were just another more complex animal descended over millions of years from earlier and simpler forms of life. The storm that followed that finding has still not subsided.

The third great insult to mankind was presented by Sigmund Freud. He demonstrated that we are not even masters in our own house, our own mind. His intensive studies through the psychoanalysis of patients showed clearly that many thoughts, motives and feelings of which we are completely unaware can be "unconscious" and yet influence our behaviors. No wonder so many people resist these assaults on their long-held and "common sense" beliefs.

"Unconscious processes" might be compared to an iceberg which towers above the surface of the ocean. We do not see its great mass hidden below the waves. Unconscious thoughts and behaviors might also be compared to events that happen in the dark of night. They do occur, but we are not aware of them.

Adventures in Human Understanding

Everyday events often reveal indirectly the presence of such underlying processes. We forget many experiences, but the fact that later we can recall them proves that these memories were not extinguished but were somewhere stored, and may often be reactivated, even if not perfectly.

On meeting a strange person we are often aware from his facial expressions, inflections of voice, gestures and posture if he doesn't like us—or we feel "instinctively" a distrust of him. Our communications may be "unconscious" to either or both of us, but a meaning has been transmitted. During an analytic psychotherapy patients often acquire "insight" into aspects of themselves of which they were previously unaware. The "unconscious" has been made conscious.

Many years ago, when I was a young psychology professor in a Western university, I and a colleague were asked to evaluate a 14-year-old boy in a nearby state who had killed his mother.

The prosecution was willing to consider an insanity plea if we could find evidence of that.

The facts of the crime were told to us as follows: The lad (I shall call him "Walden") had been admiring his new 22-caliber rifle, which, with the concurrence of his mother, he had recently received as a gift from his father.

He had placed a clip of bullets in it and was idly firing, somewhat at random, while seated on the back porch. That white rock over there. "Ping—bull's-eye." That sparrow in the tree, "Ping—bull's-eye."

His mother was hanging up washing on the clothes line. As she turned her back he sighted on her and pulled the trigger. Ping—bull's-eye.

"Mother! Mother! I didn't mean it," he shouted, rushing to her side as she fell. He was still hugging her and sobbing when a neighbor, hearing his wails, came over to investigate.

We started our evaluation expecting that we would discover a disturbed youth who displayed a record of trouble with the law and a background of child abuse—as so often is the case. The boy himself looked confused and could give no reason for shooting her. With outpourings of tears he steadfastly maintained that he loved her dearly, a statement with which the friends and neighbors agreed. We could find no record of trouble with his mother or evidence of child abuse by her. The two apparently had an affectionate and constructive parent–child relationship.

Some of the people we talked with thought it just might be a careless accident. However, the prosecutor focused on Walden's admission that he had sighted on her for some time before actually pulling the trigger. It could hardly be just an accident. Was it due to some secret, malevolent hatred, or perhaps a temporary lapse into insanity?

We began a thorough psychological evaluation: His school records, observations by his teachers, in-depth interviews with him, measures of his mental ability (the Stanford-Binet) and personality analyses, like the Rorschach Ink Blot test.

The net result: Nothing, absolutely nothing which would suggest a mental deficiency, a pathological personality or a mental insanity. We could conclude only that he was a normal boy with no evidence for either the intent or the ability to carry out a murder. Yet, why did he keep sighting on his mother before pulling the trigger?

The living situation of the family suggested more possibilities to us. His mother and father had recently been separated, and, for their own family reasons, his father had moved out of the house to a rural cabin in the nearby forest. The boy remained with his mother, while a sister, several years older, was living with the father. We resisted the temptation to apply a Freudian "Oedipal" interpretation to this arrangement.

Two bits of evidence, however, warranted further investigation. Neighbors reported that the mother and father often quarreled, and that he seemed to be very harsh and rejecting toward her. When he moved out she had pleaded with him to stay.

Adventures in Human Understanding

Walden himself furnished another important point. He told us his mother had been very upset by the separation, that she cried often, sometimes saying that life was not worthwhile, and that she wished she were dead. This had been a great source of concern for Walden, who had tried to take the place of "the man in the family" and would frequently console her.

It became increasingly clear to both of us that much more was going on under the surface of this family than was apparent. The constant depression and crying informed the boy that his mother was suffering great anguish.

In our interviews with the father (and with the sister) it was also quite obvious that the father truly hated his wife, although he avoided this term in describing her. However, he seemed very relieved that he was now free of her.

A psychological understanding of the killing of his mother by Walden now becomes possible, in fact probable. But such an interpretation requires that we recognize and accept that "unconscious" communications are involved between all three, the father, the mother and the boy.

The father disliked his wife so intensely that it had to represent a true hatred, and that he most certainly had death wishes toward her. These wishes would probably never have instigated actual murderous or aggressive behavior against her. There was no record of violence or law-breaking by the father.

Walden's mother constantly fed into the boy complaints about her pain and her wish to die. By helping her to achieve that desire he would be committing an act of mercy—such as often occurs to the caretakers of a loved one, who has suffered from a long, painful and ultimately terminal illness. The underlying message to Walden from his mother was, "I suffer. I want to die. Please help me."

At the same time the unconscious message from his father was, "I want her dead. Kill her." This was tangibly reinforced when the father, with the acquiescence of the mother, bought him the 22-caliber rifle.

A summary of the unconscious messages that the boy received might be as follows: "Mother wants to die, and Father wants her to die. I should do the killing, and the gift of the gun is the means to accomplish it." None of this (except for the mother's wish) was ever transmitted directly or verbally to Walden. He would not have been aware of these at a conscious, verbal level.

He thus became the instrument for accomplishing the death wishes of his father and the suicidal wishes of his mother. In the light of all the other information we had received, no other interpretation was credible.

We reported this to the prosecutor. He was a practical, matter-of-fact man with much experience in law enforcement. He could not accept our interpretation. All this business about the "unconscious" did not make common sense. He had heard "this stuff" before from criminals who wanted to escape the consequences of justice. No, this was not a possible explanation. The shooting had to be a crime, not an accident, and there had to be a logical reason, some true resentment in Walden against his mother.

The prosecution presented its own view of the motive for the crime: Walden had probably become very angry the night before because his mother had refused to let him go to the movies.

In court, the jury was also composed of realistic, practical citizens to whom this rationale made more sense than one based on "unconscious" motives. Walden was convicted of murder and sentenced to prison. He was thus the one who suffered the consequences of the disturbed marital relationship. The parents were exonerated from any responsibility or guilt.

I was not able to follow up on this case. However, many years later, after I became a forensic consultant to other prisons, I sadly mused about Walden's probable fate. What often happens to young boys who are sent to a men's prison is not pretty. But many of them learn to protect themselves by identifying with the prison culture and its values. Of such is the next generation of hardened criminals born.

Chapter 5

The Nerd

Brenda Gilligan and Julie Buffington, eating at a side table in the school lunchroom, looked up as Goob shuffled past them.

"Why does he wear those baggy pants every day?" giggled Brenda. "Makes him look even fatter."

"Yeah," replied Julie, scooping up another spoonful of bean soup. (Bean soup was always served on Tuesdays.) "He's a real nerd. Thinks he's so smart. Always got his hand in the air when the teacher asks a question."

"Nobody likes him. But he never seems to get mad. I called him 'Pork the Dork' the other day. Wanted to see if I could get a rise outa him. He just stared and walked on," added Brenda.

"Goob" Wilkins had reached the last table in the far corner and plunked his 225 pounds down in one of the seats. The 15-year-old Sophomore, sitting by himself, looked somewhat out of place as the lunchroom buzzed with the usual noon-day crowd of teenagers.

Goob pulled out his horn-rimmed glasses and opened up a mathematics book. Everybody ignored him, and he ignored everybody else. Having established "his table," he took a wrinkled bag out of his pack, extracted a doughnut, and settled down. Oh yes, he needed a cup of hot chocolate. So shuffling back to the counter he quietly waited until every other kid there had been served before getting his lunch ticket punched. Then, retrieving the cocoa, he returned to his table. Putting two spoonfuls of sugar in the cup, he began munching the doughnut.

Goob hated the vegetables with which his stepmother filled his lunch box each day. He always threw them away. She knew he didn't like vegetables, but insisted they were "good for you." He

Adventures in Human Understanding

had learnt a long time ago that anything "good for you" didn't taste good. So on his way to school every day he stopped off at Mrs. McIntosh's Bakery and spent his meager allowance money on two sweet rolls or two doughnuts. He wolfed down the cocoa and two doughnuts while studying the afternoon's math assignment.

Mr. Gregson would be pleased that he knew the solution of the problems better than anyone else in class. In fact, last Friday Mr. Gregson had written Goodwin Wilkins's solution to a complex quadratic equation on the blackboard and praised him before the class. Nobody applauded.

The Van Buren High School, situated in an older side of town, had probably been state of the art when it was built some 50 years earlier. Now the corner bricks were worn, a few missing, and the dark-stained desks only amplified the gloom that pervaded its classrooms. The plumbing was often clogged, and the washbasins were rusty because the school board had little money for repairs. Most of the students' parents worked at the clothing mill. It produced garments for the "trade" market. Still, the halls bustled every morning with young people, who could probably get a job at the mill when they graduated.

Goob's father was a "weaver" and operated a loom. It made the same cloth every day. Three of the weavers were to be trained to become "loom fixers," a more technical and higher-paid job. "Gus" Wilkins had applied for the position, but today he had learnt that, in spite of his seniority, the names on the "Select" list didn't include his. He was deeply disappointed. It made the half-mile he had to walk to home even more depressing. Today Goodwin's stepmother, Bessie, met Gus at the door.

"Your son refused to clean up the trash in the backyard when I told him to. It's beginning to stink," Bessie announced.

"Damn it all, Goodwin," shouted his father, "how many times do I have to tell you you've got to obey your stepmother and respect her. The next time you get no allowance for a week."

Sometimes Goodwin could stand up to his father, but not often.

"She's not my mother," he countered. "My mother died a long time ago. Just 'cause you married Bessie doesn't make her my mother. I hate her."

"Listen you! Bessie's my wife, your stepmother, and you'll love her whether you like it or not. No supper for you. Go to your room." Bessie smiled.

Goodwin stomped down the stairs to the basement, slammed the door of his room, and bolted it. At least here he could have some privacy.

When his father had married Bessie she made it clear she didn't want to put up with "that brat." But since she knew Gus had married her only so there would be someone in the house to take care of his son, Bessie shut up and begrudgingly accepted her role.

When Goodwin was in the fourth grade it was Miss McFarland who started it all. She was the principal and arithmetic teacher. Had taught there almost 40 years. One day, in a moment of confusion he had printed his name on a paper, with the "d" turned around into a "b." Miss McFarland had copied it in large letters on the blackboard in front of the class "G o o b w i n W i l k i n s." The effect on him at recess time had been devastating.

"Hi, Goob. Goob the boob. Boy what a 'goob' you are," shouted his classmates. Goodwin, hiding his tears, had run back into the schoolhouse to hide. From then on everybody called him "Goob." For several years he had endured snide remarks about "Goob." After awhile he just accepted them, and the name lost some of its sting.

Now he was alone sobbing in his room. At least it was his own room. There was a cot, one chair, bookcase and dresser. On it sat a wedding picture of his father and mother taken 16 years ago. The glass on the picture was cracked, reminding him of the time he returned from school to find it on the floor. His stepmother had "cleaned" the room that day, and he suspected she had knocked it down and left it there.

Adventures in Human Understanding

His mother, Dorothy Burton, an attractive 17-year-old blonde girl, had quit school in her Junior year and married Gus. Most of the girls in that mill town married young or got a job at the mill. Few ever went to college. Although Goodwin had dreams, and his teachers had encouraged him to think it possible, there wouldn't be any money. His Dad told him not to plan on going.

He reached for the picture with the crack and stared at it while thinking back. He had been five years old when she developed pneumonia and died. She was a jolly, happy person. Goodwin could remember a few good times they had together.

He recalled sitting on her lap while she read him bedtime stories. It seemed also that his Dad cared more for him then, but he had changed since marrying Bessie a year later. They quarreled and yelled at each other frequently. Goodwin would retreat to his basement room and wait until the shouting stopped before coming upstairs again. So it had been now for almost ten years.

Sadly he put the picture frame back on the dresser. Laying down, he thought about his world. He could see no hope. Ignored at home, rejected in school, nobody except two of the teachers paid any attention to him. Why should he go on? He had heard so many disparaging, insulting remarks over the years he was beginning to believe them.

The words of belittling classmates rang in his ears. "You're just a nerd, a dumb dork, a fatty. Get lost."

Even his angry father spoke that way at times. "You'll never amount to anything. When I was your age I had to work in the mill. You're wasting all this time in school."

Once, in a more kindly mood, he had increased Goodwin's weekly allowance from a dollar and a half to two dollars. That was because of the small raise the union had gotten at the mill.

A black mood increasingly overwhelmed Goodwin's thoughts. "Maybe I am no good. Everybody seems to think so. Perhaps they're right. I'll never amount to anything. Nobody cares."

The Nerd

The more he thought this way, the more he became convinced of his utter worthlessness. Maybe it would be better in the next world. Perhaps he would find his real mother there. The thought of it was attractive.

Another week, a deeper depression. He skipped two days of school. Spent the time wandering around in the nearby woods.

"I wonder why Goodwin missed school last week," observed Mr. Gregson. "Perhaps I'd better call his parents."

But then there were so many papers to grade. He forgot to call. Besides, the boy returned the first of the week and everything seemed O.K. The teacher, however, did note that Goodwin did not speak much or raise his hand in class as he had usually done.

During the long hours he spent alone in his room Goodwin was beginning to reach a decision. When nobody was around he often talked to himself.

"I feel terrible. Why do I feel so miserable? All the other kids seem to like living. Not me. Nobody would care whether I lived or died. Maybe I could just die. The quickest way would be to get a gun out of Dad's collection. Yes! That would be the way. If the other kids knew they made me do it, maybe they'd feel a little sorry. No! None of them would feel sorry. I could take that old revolver Dad is so proud of. Could get it after he's gone to work. He wouldn't even miss it. Bessie would be glad when I'm gone. She's always hated me. And those big shots, like 'Flash' O'Malley, 'Mitch' Shrider and the other football players would have to find somebody else to pick on."

Flash, who had won many games for Van Buren High, was a hero to the whole school. Girls clustered around him and everybody sought his company. Tall, well-built and handsome, Flash was everything Goodwin would like to have been. He laughed and told jokes. But when Goodwin was close by a mean streak in him seemed to come out.

"Hi, Nerd. You still around?"

Adventures in Human Understanding

Being put down by his "hero" hurt more than from anybody else. This convinced Goodwin more than ever that he was utterly no good and worthless in this world.

The thought about getting his father's old revolver and shooting himself went round and round in his brain. Just put it to your head: Point, bang! The idea was almost pleasurable.

Monday morning. Bessie had gone shopping. His father was at the mill. Grabbing his lunch sack, Goodwin had headed toward school. Then, deciding he couldn't face those kids again, he had walked back and quietly sat immersed in a black fog. Slowly his thoughts began to jell.

"I can do it tonight. They'd hear the gun go off. That will jar them. At least then they'll have to pay attention to me. It'll be in the newspaper. I'll be important in this town, even if it's for only one day. They'll all read about it." He could just see the *Morning Tribune*: "Goodwin Wilkins Kills Self."

The more he thought about it, the more he focused on Dad's gun. Goodwin could almost feel holding it. After he pulled the trigger he wouldn't feel pain any more (or anything else). But which gun should he take?

Gus was very proud of his gun collection. It held only a few pieces because he couldn't afford more. The antique revolver had been inherited from his grandfather who claimed it had belonged to the outlaw Billy the Kid. Also included was a 9 mm Smith and Wesson automatic, a 30-caliber Springfield for deer hunting (which came from the days when Gus as a young man had served in the National Guard), a double-barreled shotgun (for duck hunting), and his greatest pride, a 9 mm Intertech AP9.

Gus had saved for more than a year to buy this splendid weapon. Goodwin knew it was like the one that had been used by the killers at Columbine High School. When other people were calling those killers "cowards," Goodwin hadn't said anything, but he had admired them and felt they were really heroes.

The gun cabinet had been "rescued" from a second-hand store and proudly refurbished with dark stain. It stood in the dining room. About five feet tall, its glass door was kept locked. Goodwin knew that his father hid the key in the top dresser drawer in their bedroom.

"I don't want you messing around with my guns. You stay out of that cabinet," his father had admonished.

Every fall his dad went deer hunting with some buddies. They would take a day's leave from the mill on Friday, head into the hills, and spend the weekend hunting, drinking beer and exchanging dirty jokes.

Goodwin knew that some of the other kids in his school were often taken hunting by their fathers, taught gun safety, and encouraged to get a junior hunting license. He had approached his father once.

"Dad. Could you take me hunting with you this year?"

"No, Son, you'd only be in the way. I don't want to spend my time watching after you." Goodwin knew it was futile to argue. He never asked again.

And now it made no difference. While Bessie was in town shopping, he sneaked the key to the gun cabinet from his folks' dresser drawer, pocketed the old revolver and some shells, carefully re-locked the cabinet and put the key back in the drawer. The gun was hidden under his bed. Tomorrow morning he would do it. Having made up his mind, a feeling of peace descended over Goodwin's tortured brain. Exhausted, he lay down and closed his eyes.

Although seemingly asleep, he was restless, moving from one side of the bed to the other. Something was stirring deeply within him. All of a sudden he sat up in the bed. The room was filled with a strange light. Was he dreaming or was he really awake? Was the light real, or only his imagination? The light seemed to emanate from a figure standing near the bed. He rubbed his eyes.

"Goodwin. Goodwin."

Was he hearing a real voice Or only a dream voice? He felt confused and struggled to decide. Couldn't make up his mind.

"Goodwin, Dear. Don't you know me? Don't you remember?" That voice was strangely familiar. He must have heard it before. Maybe a long time ago. The white figure came closer.

He looked up at it, now very close. Suddenly a burst of recollection overwhelmed him. With a flood of tears he shouted, "Mama. Mama."

"Yes, Dear. I am your mother, Dorothy. I am here because you need me. Can I hold you?"

He reached his arms toward the figure, and the figure of a fair-haired young woman wrapped hers around him. He felt somehow that he was no longer fifteen years old. He was a 3-year-old boy being rocked by his Mama. Although at times he had dreamt of such an occasion, he hadn't been held this way for many years.

Goodwin felt overwhelmingly happy. His hell of anguish melted away midst a heaven of ecstasy.

"Dear. Mother knows you have a problem, a very serious one. You have been trying to solve it for a long time."

"Yes, Mama. And now I'm with you. Can I stay here?"

His mother didn't answer at first. Then after a long pause she gently said, "You will have to decide that. But first you must see some things before you judge."

Goodwin wondered what he must see—and what he must decide. But he continued to listen.

"We will take a trip. There is a small boat outside, and the lake is not very large. Come!"

Taking him by the hand, she led him out of the house. He was amazed to see a shimmering body of water outside instead of the street in front of his home. Together they walked toward a sandy beach where sat a small row-boat. Climbing in, they pushed off.

"Where are we going, Mama. What must I see?"

"You must see some people, my little Son, many people—and a very important, powerful person."

"But Mama, who are these people, and where are they?"

"All in good time. But you must row now. There is only an hour left—before the morning sun will come and wash this away."

Goodwin was puzzled by his mother's remark, but he rowed briskly, pulling the oars with all the energy his pudgy little arms could muster. A sandy beach fronting a thick green forest appeared dimly in the distance. It was obviously an island. He stared at it in wonderment. As they approached its shores he noticed movement. A multitude of people were shouting, waving their arms, and running up and down the beach.

"Who are those people, and why are they shouting," asked Goodwin?"

"Pull up closer and look at them carefully," replied his mother.

"They look very scared, Mama. And many of them are crying. Why are they crying?"

"They are begging for their lives."

"But why? Are their lives in danger? Does someone want to hurt them?"

His mother looked at Goodwin very thoughtfully before replying.

"There is an important person on this island. He is very powerful, but he doesn't know how important he is. He has the power of life or death over all of them."

Adventures in Human Understanding

"But Mama. Is he a mean, bad person. Does he want to kill all these people?'

"No, my Son. He isn't bad or mean. He just doesn't recognize how much they need him. He doesn't know that without his help they will all die."

"Can't we find him? Can't we explain to him, convince him to save their lives? They look like such nice people. And see those two boys and the girl in the front row. The cute little boy with the curly hair must be two years old and the other, the boy that's bigger, would be fun to play with. The blonde girl is pretty. Maybe she's old enough to go to school."

More questions came to Goodwin's mind. "Do you mean they and all the others will die? We've just got to help them. Who is that important person, and where can we find him?"

"We have to return now to where we started this journey, Son. Please row us back home," said Mother.

Goodwin was puzzled when she spoke no more but just pointed to the boat. He had to pull very hard on the oars because of a strong head wind. It seemed a long time before the beach appeared from which they started.

He was tired, very tired. There were so many questions on his mind, but he was getting befogged again. He needed to sleep. His mother almost had to carry the little boy the last few steps. Tucking him in his bed, and kissing him "Good Night," she melted away. Goodwin was soon fast asleep.

It was morning, but still dark, when Goodwin aroused and threw off the covers. He had to go to the bathroom. Returning, he lay on the bed and pulled up the blanket. He wanted to go back to sleep, but his mind remained active, vigorously active.

"Did I really see my mother? Where was the island we visited? And who were all those people? She had said a very important person had life or death power over them. And that he wasn't mean or cruel. He just didn't realize his power. Who was that person? Where could I find him?" Goodwin drowsed off again.

While still in a half-sleepy state he became aware of the light once more. The same soft voice spoke again to him.

"My Son. You can see that most important person now if you will look out the dining-room window."

This seemed to make no sense to Goodwin, but it was the voice of his Mother. He knew she wouldn't mislead him. So, struggling out of his bed, he tiptoed up the stairs to the dining room, around the oval table with its chairs, and past the gun cabinet. He remembered that he had to do something important about it, but right now he couldn't remember just what.

Next, he walked over to the far window that looked out onto the driveway. There was only a dim light in the room. The window had an unusual glare. Goodwin stared out, but it was dark. He couldn't make out the driveway or the garage.

The light in the room brightened. He stared at the window in astonishment. It had turned into a mirror. In it he could see the face of a teenage boy. It appeared strange to him.

Suddenly a flash of recognition crossed his mind. The features looked just like those which he saw every morning while washing his face. Frightened, he rushed down the stairs, quietly closing and locking his door. The white light became strong, and once more he saw the image of his mother smiling at him.

"My Son. Now you know who that most important person is, the one with the power of life or death over all those people."

Even though the covers were warm, Goodwin was shaking from head to foot. He couldn't believe what he had observed.

"But mother, who are all those people, and who are the little children in front?"

It seemed like forever before his mother replied, "Those people are your descendants. The three little ones in front are my grandchildren to be—your children. And those behind, begging for their lives, are their children and their children's children. It could go back for hundreds of years, the many descendants of Goodwin Wilkins. They will live if that person in the mirror, you, does not kill them off."

Goodwin burst into an uncontrollable fit of crying. He hid his head under the covers so that his parents upstairs would not hear him. It was all very clear now. He had never thought of himself as powerful and important to so many people.

The light was gradually fading from the room.

"Don't leave me, Mother. I need you." From far away he heard her voice.

"Please don't kill my grandchildren and our descendants, Dear Son. Let that person in the mirror live, so they too can live." Then the voice faded away.

Goodwin felt as if a huge burden had been lifted from him. He fell back on the bed in a deep slumber from which he awakened only to hear his father's voice. It seemed warmer and more friendly than usual.

"Goodwin. Time to get up. Breakfast will be ready in ten minutes."

The next few days Goodwin felt a calming of the angry tension which had filled him. He knew he was important for those who were yet to come. And he understood his mother's love. He also felt now he would never kill himself. That had been settled. However, the teasing from his classmates continued and added to his reservoir of hatred. But what next?

He kept thinking of Flash, Mitch, and the other football players who had tormented him. He wanted to have one more good look at them. He would go to the Friday afternoon game.

The Nerd

He knew that his very appearance would probably set off another round of derision, but he would have to take a chance. Seating himself inconspicuously behind the end zone, he huddled down. Those sitting beside him ignored him, and he paid no attention to them.

Goodwin was in agonizing conflict. The brilliant runs by Flash, who carried passes for long gains in yardage, stirred him. He admired and wanted to cheer. Then his memories of the many put-downs by Flash would arise. More feelings of hatred reached awareness.

He turned his attention to Mitch, the quarterback. Mitch had been even rougher than Flash. In Mitch, Goodwin found nothing to admire. Late in the game the center, Charley Edmunds, passed the ball to Mitch, who faded back to pass. Suddenly a tackle from Bowers Grove, of the opposing team, broke through and slammed his 250 pounds against Mitch. Mitch fell to the ground and didn't get up. A mountain of "Oh"s from the crowd reverberated through the stadium. Almost everybody but Goodwin stood up. Mitch didn't move. Finally a stretcher crew came running onto the field, and Mitch was hauled away to the hospital.

Goodwin thought, "That's one bastard that's got what he deserves." He left the football game feeling rather pleased.

In the next few days a new mood began to steal over him. Something was fermenting in the corridors of his mind. No more despair, just an inside rage. He no longer felt helpless. The more Goodwin thought of the ridicule heaped on him over the years, the madder he got.

In the privacy of his room he could drowse on his bed while mulling over delicious thoughts in his mind.

"Those sons-of-bitches, those dirty sons-of-bitches. How many other guys have they bullied? They don't deserve to live. Somebody should have the guts to waste them. Then they'd never again be able to inflict such misery on others. Somebody's got to fight for the little guys. Who? Me? Why not me? If I don't, and nobody else does, they'll keep right on sneering and humiliating

Adventures in Human Understanding

the rest of us. They're no better than Hitler and the Nazis. Damn it all. I'll do it. I'll show the world they can't get away with it. And anybody else who abuses and hurts innocent kids. I'll be their champion—but how do I go about it?"

Having reached a decision, Goodwin's fury momentarily subsided. He turned to planning just how he would annihilate those villains. He threw himself so completely into the images of destruction that he was no longer in the reality of his own room.

"Let's see. That old revolver of Dad's is not enough. I can't get more than one or two of them before the police come. I'll need to take the 9 mm Intertech. That's got some power. I can get a lot more of them."

By now he had forgotten all about his children and those other descendants, whose lives he was supposed to protect. Vaguely he realized he would probably be arrested and sent to prison.

"So, maybe I'll get caught and charged with a crime. But what is my crime?" Once again rage conquered any misgivings.

"Ridding the world of sons-of-bitches that bring misery to innocent people like me. They ought to give me a medal for that. I don't care if I go to jail. I will have done a good deed for all mankind. That's the kind of people the world needs. A few who will stand up for right—even if they personally get punished. I can save a lot of other students from being hurt."

Goodwin focused his attention now toward accomplishing his goal. Before his dream with his mother he had felt weak. He thought then of himself as a helpless victim. Now he felt strong. As the avenger he was no longer depressed. It was as if bursts of new energy were rushing through his veins. He thought no longer of suicide, of self-murder. Now he dared to hate others. He was important. He was powerful. And "By God," they would respect him.

"If I can catch them as they come out of the building and head toward the practice field maybe I can get most of them: Flash, Mitch, Charley and the others on the team."

The Nerd

As he thought of watching them emerge from the school, he could almost feel himself pulling the trigger of the Intertech. He laughed. What a wonderful feeling of controlling one's world. His time was coming.

But now to business. He must not slip up. "Maybe if I made a bomb, one of those pipe bombs, and exploded it in the front of the school, everybody will get scared and rush out the back door. Then I can get more of them, including those smart-assed girls who made fun of me."

Goodwin couldn't figure out just how to build a bomb, but he thought maybe "www.bomb.com" on the Internet might provide the information. There were a number of websites that responded. They all offered historical information on the development of bombs, those dropped from airplanes, etc. He couldn't find one that gave the specific instructions he needed to construct one. So reluctantly he decided he must act without waiting to find out. Maybe if he turned on the fire alarm …

He went up to the dresser in his parents' bedroom and again retrieved the key for the gun cabinet. Unlocking it, he secured the Intertech—folded his coat over it (in case Bessie unexpectedly returned), and quickly went downstairs. After locking the door he hid the gun under the bed.

Admiringly he thought, "Isn't it a beauty? No wonder Dad paid so much for it."

Goodwin had watched his father once shooting it on the firing range, and was amazed at how many bullets it could handle in a few seconds. Two clips, twenty shells.

"That's plenty of power," he decided. He was ready. He would do the job. Relaxing on the bed, he began methodically planning the details. It was just like solving a mathematics problem.

He had to sneak the gun into the school and get it into his locker (No. 218, second floor). If he arrived late the teachers and students would be in class. The halls would be empty. Of course, he might

Adventures in Human Understanding

run into Mr. Gimbel, the janitor. But if the gun were not in sight he could take a chance on that.

Nobody must see him with a gun when he was going to school. How could he hide it? He thought of his old gray raincoat with the deep pockets. It looked rainy today. Most of the kids would be wearing bright yellow raincoats, which were popular.

Goodwin hated that coat. He had asked his father if he could get a new designer coat like the other students had. At that moment Bessie had cut in.

"No need to waste all that money. I can get him one at Goodwill for less than half as much." His father had agreed.

Marching him into the Goodwill store she had found this shabby-looking, gray one. It was the only one that fit him. So now he went to school dressed different than the rest of the students. Goodwin hated wearing it. However, he recalled reading that the young gunmen at the Columbine School had worn long, black coats. Maybe this one would do after all.

He took one clip of cartridges, inserted them in the gun, put it in the coat right pocket and slipped the other clip in the left pocket. Then with a mixture of determination and misgivings, he set off for school.

It was nine-thirty when he arrived. The classrooms were busy, but the halls were deserted. Quickly he scooted up to the second floor, dialed his lock number, and hung the coat inside. There was no sign of Mr. Gimbel.

Goodwin attended his other classes throughout the day, but his mind was so engrossed with rehearsing plans that he was almost startled when the four o'clock bell sounded. The halls rapidly filled as the students poured out.

He knew that almost all of them met the buses in front. The boys in the football team, however, would go to the locker room, suit up, and emerge about fifteen minutes later out the back door, which led to the playing field.

He had planned his next step very carefully. At the back of the playing field there was a clump of bushes. He got his coat, went out the back door quickly and lay down behind the clump. From there he had a good view of the door, not much more than 20 yards away. The land behind him sloped down toward the river.

Laying on his belly, he peered out over the clump of bushes. He held the pistol straight out with both hands—as he had seen the police do on television.

The back door of the school building opened. Two boys clad in football clothes emerged. Goodwin held his fire until a third one appeared. He was certain this was Flash. Then he squeezed the trigger with all his might; the shells rapidly discharged. Bang! Bang! Bang! At a distance they might have sounded like firecrackers. But to Goodwin they were the most satisfying explosions he had ever heard. He saw two of the figures go down, blood spurting out. The last one, Flash, staggered before he fell.

Screams could be heard all over the neighborhood. Several boys, just coming out the back door, realized something was wrong. Hastily retreating, they slammed the door. Voices were heard yelling. "Somebody's got a gun." "Get out of here." "Call the police." The starting of many cars in the side lot, however, drowned out much of this clamor.

Goodwin felt an enormous sense of exhilaration. He was flying over the scene like a destroying angel. He could no longer restrain himself. His dreams were coming true. Jumping to his feet he began hollering at the prone bodies in front of the school back door.

"You sons-of-bitches. It's me, Goob. You didn't think I'd ever dare, did you. You'll never bully any more good kids. You're going to hell. D'ya hear me. It's Goob. Goob, who you've been kicking around for years."

He was exploding with a devastating blast, fed by enormous wells of stifled rage. No thought of consequence. No holding back. It was everything he wanted, the eruption like that of Vesuvius blowing its top and with lava-rivers of hate destroying everything in their path. For a minute his fury continued this way. Then, the clip of cartridges was exhausted. Goodwin was exhausted. His world seemed to stand still. Although screams, shouts and the wailing of police sirens besieged the air, he could hear none of it. Momentarily he was like a mute stone statue, frozen in time and space.

Slowly, within a few seconds, thought, reason and feelings returned.

"My God! What have I done? I gotta get away right now." In a few minutes the police and others would be converging on him. Dashing down the incline toward the river he soon put several trees between him and the gory event behind the school. If he could run fast enough along the river bank, perhaps he could escape. No one could see him down by the river. He thought of jumping in a deep hole and drowning himself. But he didn't want to die—even if it meant spending the rest of his life in prison.

He spotted the big eddy at the bend of the river. The river here, before making a sharp turn, swirled around and around. He must get rid of this damned pistol. Throwing it as hard as he could, he noted with some relief that it landed in the middle of the big fishing hole. He knew the eddy was at least 20 feet deep. Rushing away, he glanced back and saw the gun sinking. It was heavy. It would go to the bottom. He had fled only a few steps when he recalled he was still carrying the extra clip in his coat pocket. He must return and throw it, too, into the surging waters. Quick! People would be coming. He fumbled in his pocket. No, it must be in the other one. He could barely hear the shouts of students now, but the pulsating police sirens struck terror to his soul.

He wondered whether his fingerprints would show if they found the gun. But no! That was impossible. It would rot at the bottom of the river for many years. Now he must get home and hide. He must hope that Bessie and his father were still away. He had to sneak in the back door, rush downstairs, lock his own door, go to bed and, shivering all over, pull the covers over his head.

Once before, when he was five years old, he had stolen a candy bar at Mr. Pyett's drugstore. Stuffed it in his pants pocket and ran home. His father found him huddled in bed and had beaten him severely. It was the same now—only much worse.

Gasping, panting and sobbing he felt an enormous sense of coldness. Maybe he was dying. No longer did he think of what he had just done. He was returning to the folds of his infancy. He didn't feel fifteen years old. He didn't feel five years old, or three years old. He didn't feel at all. Only that he was immersed in a cloud of darkness. Mercifully sleep took over. He was dead to the world.

It was hours later when his coma was disturbed.

"Goodwin! Goodwin! Can you hear me?"

He didn't understand at first. He rubbed his eyes while waving his hands futilely in the air. He poured every last bit of his energy into trying to focus on that voice. Finally, he recognized it.

"Mama. Oh My God, Mama. I'm so glad you've come." Another flood of tears as he desperately reached out, trying to make contact with the vision in front of him.

"I've done a bad, bad, thing Mama. I don't know what to do. Will they hang me? Will they send me to prison for the rest of my life?"

Why wasn't his mother more disturbed? How could she stand there in front of him and not be horrified? Surely she must know. Or did she? Goodwin felt he had to tell her. He must tell her. Perhaps if he confessed maybe she would forgive him, even if the rest of the world didn't.

"My Son. You did what you needed to do. You couldn't have done differently."

Was this his mother, his gentle mother who abhorred all violence? Could she really speak this way?"

She continued, "Do you see your coat over there hanging in the closet? Reach into its pocket."

Adventures in Human Understanding

Goodwin threw the covers off and slowly moved to the closet. Putting his hand into the left pocket he felt something hard. Grasping it and pulling it out he saw that he was holding a clip of cartridges.

"Mama. How can this be? I threw that clip away into the river."

"Reach in the other pocket, Dear."

Totally bewildered, he did and pulled out the pistol. He shook his head in total amazement.

"But Mama, I threw that in the river too. After I had shot all those fellows. I watched it sink. What's it doing in my coat pocket?"

His mother sat in the chair in front of him. Reaching arms out, she pulled him close to her. He felt again like a little boy, but he knew he really was fifteen, a high school student.

"My Son, you were so loaded with hatred that you needed to eliminate all those who had been hurting you. Yes, indeed, you needed to get rid of that huge reservoir of anger buried in you. It was like an infection, poisoning your soul. Unless you did what you needed to do it would have stayed there until it destroyed you. But Goodwin, you did it the right way. You did it through a fantasy in your dreams. You carried it through inside you. Then you didn't have to do it on the outside—where it would have destroyed you and many others. This whole experience happened inside your mind."

From the depths of hell, Goodwin's heart jumped to the peaks of elation.

"You mean I didn't really kill anyone? That I just thought it, imagined it?"

"Much more than that, my Son. If you had only thought it, only imagined it, it would have been just thoughts. You had to live it and experience it with all those feelings of rage. It needed to be resolved within your own self. You had to feel all that hatred and experience all those killings. But you did it while you were still asleep. You remember that time when you were so frightened of the monster? You really saw that monster. And you really felt scared, deathly fearful for your life. But the monster was in your dream—just as the killings were in your dream."

"But Mother, isn't there some way I can make up for it?" I'm not angry anymore. But I still feel guilty for even having thought about killing those fellows."

"Yes, there is, Son, but you must find it for yourself. If you do, you will learn how to be a happy man."

The light around the vision faded. Then it was gone. Goodwin was too exhausted to even protest her leaving. He fell back into a profound slumber. As he took Mom's hand he recalled their previous adventure when she had saved his life—and those of his descendants. It didn't seem to be quite the same now. In the first place he didn't feel three years old. He knew clearly that he was fifteen. And second, there was some unpleasant feeling which was different. He didn't label it as guilt. But it might have been.

The two of them proceeded hand in hand down the street, past the school building toward where the houses were smaller, dingier and generally unpainted. They stopped before one of the poorest ones. The sun was almost overhead. On the bare, brown and ill-kept lawn was a small boy. He was holding a strap which was attached to the collar of a little black and white puppy terrier. The little dog was yelping, trying to run away. The boy was laughing and yanking the strap back and forth.

"Mom. Why is that boy mean to the puppy? Doesn't he know that it is in pain?"

"Just keep watching, Son."

As he continued to observe, he saw the boy pick up a big stick and start beating the puppy. Now it was howling in pain and in terror.

"Stop it! Stop it! I don't want to watch. The boy's being mean," furiously shouted Goodwin, clenching his fists. "I hate him. He's one of those people we need to get rid of. Can I stop him?"

Adventures in Human Understanding

"Not right now, Son. I want you to see another scene first."

Goodwin was puzzled. Why didn't she want to stop the beating? He had a feeling as if the sun were moving backward, back to the east, and it was in the morning.

"Where are we going, Mom?"

She took him by the hand and led him toward the back door of the house. Opening a creaking old door, they entered. They seemed to be standing in a small living room.

Curled on a dingy faded-brown couch was a small boy looking at a picture book. Suddenly the front door burst open, and a large, burly man in the working clothes of a mill worker appeared.

The boy, startled, jumped out of the chair and tried to run toward a door leading to a hallway.

"Come here, Michael," the large man roared in a menacing voice. Slowly, timorously, and with an awareness of what was to come, the boy obeyed.

"You left your tricycle in the middle of the garage. It hit the fender of my car when I came it. Left a dent. How many times must I teach you?"

The boy knew that his dad's ancient Oldsmobile had many dents in its rusty fenders. Why should one more make such a difference? But he wouldn't dare mention that.

The man grabbed the boy's head and began beating him with fists on the head and back.

"Please, Daddy. Please. I won't ever do it again."

Desperately Michael struggled, trying to get away. He wasn't strong enough. Flailing around, he was screaming with fear and pain.

"Oh God. Help me. Mama. Where are you?"

The wilder Michael twisted back and forth, the more violent the red-faced father continued beating.

"When you need to be disciplined, don't you ever invoke the name of The Lord or expect your mother to intervene. For that you're really going to get it now." The blows became more frequent. Michael's parents were very devout church-goers.

Finally, as if exhausted, the big man let go of the boy's arm and stomped out of the room. The small lad, sobbing, ran behind the large sofa and huddled there—hiding.

Goodwin was furious.

"Mother, what a terrible thing to do to a little boy, just a helpless little guy. That man should be beaten himself, or maybe killed. He doesn't deserve to have a son."

Goodwin was so angry he tightened up all his muscles, striking out with clenched fists as if he were really hitting the man. Finally he quieted down, still shaking with rage.

"Did you notice who the boy was?" softly inquired his mother.

"Who? Just some boy called Michael. I haven't seen him before."

"Oh yes, you have," replied mother. "Did you notice his tan shirt and the blue jeans?"

Goodwin's face lit up. Suddenly it was if a new understanding had arrived.

"Why, it's the boy who was beating the dog. The one who made me so mad watching him do it."

"That's right, Son. Now you know why he beat his little dog. He was beaten by his father. His father's hatred was transferred to him. He took out on that puppy the same anger that his father took on him. Hatred and being mean is like a disease. One gets it from being mistreated. Then one passes it on to another—especially if he is small and helpless, like Michael was at that time."

Adventures in Human Understanding

Goodwin was so astonished he sat down. Never before had he thought about this problem.

"But Mother, how we can we know the good guys from the bad guys?" He was remembering all the cowboy movies he had seen at the Roxy. The bad guys wore the black hats and fought dirty. The good guys always wore white hats and fought fair. You had to know right from wrong, and which guys were on the right side.

Goodwin's mother continued. "You said you wanted to beat up on the boy when he beat the puppy. You would be acting just like Michael's father. Do you still want to?"

Goodwin was getting more confused by the minute.

"But Mother, I don't know that guy. But when I saw the way his father was beating him, I didn't feel angry at him anymore. I felt sorry for him."

"You mean you feel sorry for a mean guy when you know what or who made him mean?"

"I can feel sorry for him when he's not mean—like beating the puppy. And I feel sorry for him when a mean father is beating him. Who is he? I don't know him."

"Oh yes, you do. You know him well. I guess you just didn't know his real name was Michael. You called him by another name. Let's see him when he's in high school."

The world spun around. It was like a fast forward on the VCR. Goodwin often used the fast forward when he didn't want to watch all the advertising. The scene changed. It was now a familiar-looking school building. Somebody was coming out.

"Mother. Mother. It's Mitch, Mitch Shrider. He's the one who's the meanest of all. He's been teasing me for years."

With a sinking feeling Goodwin suddenly remembered that he had planned to kill Mitch tomorrow. In fact, he was the one he wanted to waste most of all—Mitch and Flash.

His mother continued.

"Yes. I know. You've always hated him. Do you still hate him?" Goodwin slowly shook his head, but it took an effort. He wasn't sure now. He wasn't sure of anything now.

"Yeah that's true. But I didn't know his father used to beat him. Is that where he got to being mean—mean to me?"

Mother paused a moment before looking at him with that wise smile. "What do you think? You said you hated him when he was beating on the puppy. And you didn't hate him when his father was beating him. He wasn't the bad guy then; he was the good guy. And I know you hate him in school. Well, do you hate him now, or not?"

This was a real tough problem for Goodwin. What was right, and what was wrong?

"Well, I had been hating him—so much I wanted to kill him. Now, when I know where he learned to be mean I don't hate him, at least very much. I guess I couldn't shoot him now. Can't we get the meanness out of people? If they hate because they've been hated, does it have to go on?" Inside Goodwin was waging a battle with himself.

"Maybe there's a way," replied his mother.

Goodwin broke down. Sobbing, he felt so confused. All those mean guys that he was going to eliminate. Maybe every one of them could have been hurt, put down, humiliated, like himself. Now he didn't know whether he would be a hero or a bad guy. His mother put her arm around his shoulder. It felt good. Once more he seemed to be a small child.

The wise, soft voice continued. "Perhaps we hate other people, maybe even other countries, because we don't understand them. When they do things to hurt us, to humiliate us, we don't understand how they got that way. Maybe if we understood them better we wouldn't have to hate them."

Adventures in Human Understanding

Goodwin had calmed down and was beginning to think more clearly. His high intelligence, that which made him first in the mathematics class, began to swing into high gear. What was the solution for this problem?

"Mom. Can I do something to get rid of hate, in me and in them?" He looked at her pleadingly. Everything she said seemed to make sense.

"Didn't you have a friend once, when you were in the fifth grade, who went to bat for you?"

"How did you know that, Mom? That was after you had gone."

"There are many things we don't understand, many mysteries. But I know so much about you—and I will always love you."

Goodwin began remembering. "It was in the fifth grade. His name was Jeremy. When the other kids made fun of me, he wasn't one of them. He made me feel respected. Once, when I forgot my lunch he shared his sandwich. I always felt sad when his family moved away."

"You mean that when you felt respected you liked him, and couldn't hate him as you did the others?"

Another light seemed to have just been turned on in Goodwin's brain. Now he understood what he lacked. Maybe it was also what lay hidden in others—the feeling of being respected. Maybe he could make a bigger impact in the world this way than by killing his enemies? He opened his eyes. Where was his mother? Was she just a dream? The dawn was just beginning to peep in through the shades. Today would be a most important one. Reaching into his dresser drawer he retrieved a small tin can, extracted its contents, and stuffed it into his pocket.

Classes quit early this day in order that the student body could have a general meeting. Student President Jim McNeil called the meeting together, and a few routine motions were passed. One of

The Nerd

the girls made a small speech noting that Mitch Wozinsky was in St. Mary's Hospital, had to have an operation for a broken rib and would be confined there for perhaps a week. She moved that the student body authorize the Treasurer to allocate funds to buy a large bouquet of flowers showing the school's appreciation and that everybody sign a "Get Well" card.

"All those in favor raise their right hand," declared President McNeil. "Opposed, the same." Agreement was unanimous.

"Carried," he announced. "Is there any other business someone wants to bring up?"

Goodwin had been thinking almost all night. He had made a decision. This was the moment he was waiting for. He had remembered his friend Jeremy Sloan. Jeremy was large for his age, and when a number of the older boys had started bullying him Jeremy had faced them down and made them lay off. Goodwin always remembered that experience. Somebody cared, and he was grateful. Jeremy had made in Goodwin a friend for life simply by giving him a simple protective gesture, unasked for but meaningful. Maybe Jeremy knew the secret of winning friends.

Now the time had come for him to make his move, one he had spent almost all night planning. Dared he do it? Goodwin raised his hand and signaled to Jim McNeil. President McNeil announced, "The chair recognizes Goob Wilkins. What do you have to say, Goob?"

Jim had been well coached in parliamentary protocol by the debate teacher, Mr. Coulter. He knew how to conduct a meeting. That is why he had been elected Student Body President.

Goodwin stood up.

Some cries rang through the study hall. "Sit down, nerd."

"Shut him up, the smart aleck" and "Down with fatso."

Jim pounded his gavel. "There will be order. Goob has the floor."

Adventures in Human Understanding

Goodwin's heart jumped up in his throat. He almost sat down, but mustering all the composure he could manage, he announced in loud, clear terms: "Mitch has put our school on the map, what with him producing the winning touchdowns in the championship game." Goodwin glanced at Flash. "Him and Flash."

"Mitch will appreciate our remembering him. But flowers won't be of much help. I heard my parents talking last night. Mitch's dad is a weaver at the mill. Business has been bad, and the mill is firing a number of the weavers. The Union said that a lot of men had more seniority. Mitch's father would have to go. His parents don't have a lot of money. Why don't we do something that would really help Mitch?"

The hubbub quieted down. It was quiet. Flash, who had been lounging back with his long legs hanging over the desk, suddenly sat up and wearing a puzzled look on his face stared at Goodwin.

Goodwin continued. "I move we set up a fund to help pay for Mitch's operation. It may not pay all the bills, but it would help. If each of us put some money into it, and then we organized a committee that contacted the downtown storekeepers, I bet we could raise a lot. I'll start it out by putting in five dollars." Reaching in his pocket Goob extracted a handful of dollar bills, and deposited them on the table in front.

There was a deafening silence. The student body was stunned. How come this nerd was standing there and taking the leadership role in a project that had never occurred to them? There was a murmur of approval. A few clapped. Then more.

Jim McNeil announced, "Is there a second?" There were several shouts of "Second." "All in favor raise their hand." Every hand was raised. "Carried," he announced with a smile on his face.

"Goob, you started this. Would you take the responsibility to chair a committee to plan for raising the money?" Goob nodded. "Then I want five volunteers." A number of hands went up, including Brenda's.

"Meeting is adjourned."

The Nerd

Everybody left feeling good. Goob got more attention in the next ten minutes than he had had in years. He was glowing all over when he started home.

The next morning he noticed many students were looking quizzically at him, as if somehow they hadn't seen him before.

At noon he went to the lunch room and sat down at his corner table. Before he could open his lunch sack, Flash and Charley Edmunds sidled over looking somewhat uncomfortable.

"Hey Goob, can we join you?" mumbled Charley

Flash was more straightforward. "You're not such a nerd after all. That's a damned nice thing you did for Mitch." In five minutes he and Charley were talking football strategy. Goob was listening with all ears.

Flash looked him over, then said, "Ever wanted to play football, Goob?"

Nobody had ever suggested this to him. It was what he always wanted to do.

Flash continued. "You're big. Might play guard or tackle. You'd have to get in condition though. Too flabby. And get some of that lard off your belly."

Charley said, "Maybe he could. Why don't we ask Coach Callahan to take a look at him?"

"Good idea," agreed Flash.

The next day after school Flash and Charley escorted Goob to Coach Callahan's office.

The coach, a huge, burly man sporting an almost white moustache, was planning next year's roster. He looked up from his desk.

"I'm kinda busy now, fellows. What's on your mind?"

Adventures in Human Understanding

Flash took the lead. "Coach, we've got a friend who might be shaped into a team player by next year."

The coach recognized Goodwin. In fact he had seen this big fat boy many times in the halls but had never thought of him as football material.

"Hi Goob! You interested in becoming a football player?"

Goodwin was so overwhelmed he could hardly mumble, "Yes, sir."

Coach Callahan uttered a few "Mmms" as he looked Goodwin up and down. Noticing the eager interest on the faces of two of his best players he overcame his doubts and said appraisingly, "Maybe! Get the fat off. Build more muscle in your arms and legs. Exercise, jog. Cut out the sweets. It won't be easy."

Goob took it all in as if the Pope was quoting the Bible.

"I'll try real hard, sir."

Accustomed to quick judgments, Coach Callahan decided to take a chance.

The net result of all this was that the coach told him he had possibilities.

"Report for practice when spring training begins next March. Maybe you can try out for that vacancy left by our right guard, Greg Putnam. He graduates in June, you know." The coach dismissed him. Goodwin jogged all the way home, his head in a cloud.

The next morning he forgot to stop at the McIntosh Bakery. Raced right by it. At noon, Flash invited him to have lunch at the large table where most of the school's athletes ate. Goodwin was very hungry but excitedly enjoyed participating in all the football talk. On leaving the table he noticed that he had eaten all the vegetables in his lunch pack.

Thoughts of a Therapist: Analysis and Comment

Newspapers today are filled with reports of violence. Especially sad are those involving adolescent suicide or homicide. A very depressed youth acquires a gun, often in the home, and shoots himself—"selbstmordt" or self-murder as the Germans call it.

In another case he appears at school with a machine pistol or semi-automatic, shooting other students and teachers—often at random. Law enforcement officials appear helpless, family members are devastated and a bewildered community asks "Why?"

Frequently, the question seems unanswerable. He was a good student, quiet, did not cause trouble, and showed no prior evidence of a potential for violence. In such cases one must look into "unconscious" processes to find a rationale.

There are many approaches to psychotherapy, but "psycho-dynamically-oriented" psychologists and other such mental health practitioners specifically emphasize the role of unconscious motivations in determining unexplainable behaviors.

In the case of Goodwin, the hero of our story, "The Nerd," many motives are observable to others or within the conscious awareness of the individual. But many others are below his threshold of consciousness and not discernible. In such cases the practitioner must infer their existence, employ hypnosis, "ego-state" methods or some other variation of "psychoanalytic" therapy. How might he/she view the hero in this story?

Goodwin is a fictional character but constructed of many "pieces of persons," real-life people, whom the writer (teacher and therapist) saw in school classrooms and in the consulting treatment office. Goodwin's conflicts and motivations are typical of many young people today, as in past years.

When the story starts, this fat boy is rejected and scorned by classmates. He appears to ignore this abuse, even allowing himself to be pushed around at the lunch counter. He compensates by excelling scholastically, and his intellectual skills are demonstrated by a well-meaning teacher, Mr. Gregson, which, however, only adds to his peer rejection. We assume that underneath he is filled with much anger.

To assuage his inner feeling of loneliness he also over-eats rich food which increases his fatness. Some rejected or scorned people acquire obesity by aggressively eating at the abuser. Of such are the inner signs of repressed rage.

At home, Goodwin is confronted by a hostile stepmother, who is angry at him. She knows her husband, Gus, married her only so she could serve as a housekeeper and child-sitter for his son. We see her taking out this spite on Goodwin, enlisting Gus in her rejection of the lad.

Gus, Goodwin's father, is unhappily married to her, a great contrast from his loved first wife, Dorothy, who "abandoned" him through death. He and Bessie constantly quarrel. He cannot be a good father, let alone a support for Goodwin. At work in a monotonous job, he is overlooked for promotions, initiating more anger. It is taken out on Goodwin. Gus cannot accept the role of good father and fails to take opportunities to relate to the boy, but immerses himself in the hobby of collecting guns. Sometimes he leaves the home on brief hunting expeditions where his own anger can take the form of killing deer. There is almost nothing positive in this house for him, Bessie or Goodwin.

Miss McFarland, an obsessive-compulsive teacher, who is not interested in children, only in the "correctness" of mathematics, seizes on an early spelling mistake by Goodwin to release on him a cycle of humiliation and rejection from "cruel" classmates. His world becomes only misery. No wonder he is a time bomb waiting to explode in violence.

A defense for the deeply depressed Goodwin is to retreat from painful reality to the privacy of his room and day-dream. Such day-dreaming is not unlike the couch-relaxation "free association" of the psychoanalytic patient. His periods of half-sleep are also similar to the state of hypnosis, a twilight zone, where unconscious processes may become more overt. It is in such states where he "regresses" to childhood and accesses hidden wishes and forgotten memories. One of these is of his loving, nurturing mother whom he lost at age five. He sees her in this half-awake state as a fantasy, almost a true hallucination.

In his reverie she is a saving-angel and an inner therapist. She counters his feeling of impotence and worthlessness by showing him that his life is important both to her, her "unborn grandchildren" and their descendants. This support and new insight from within enables him to relinquish his fantasies of self-destruction. He is greatly invigorated—typical of the sequel to a successful episode of psychotherapy.

However, his basic problem, inner rage, created by the long-standing rejection of family and classmates, is not eliminated. It is still hidden within, like an unseen cancer. Soon it begins to manifest itself.

No longer feeling helpless, he becomes increasingly aware of his anger, though not as yet the magnitude of the potential violence within. As this moves to consciousness he develops a "paranoid" system which demands revenge against hostile classmates. He plans to kill them and rationalizes it as becoming a champion for all mistreated young people.

A therapeutic technique useful in cases of encapsulated trauma is to release (under hypnosis) dissociated fear, rage, guilt or other unconscious motivations. Goodwin is now showing signs of anger overtly, but neither he nor others are aware of just how really mad he is. He is like a boiler filled with steam under pressure waiting to explode. From the outside it looks the same as a similar boiler with little or no pressure within. Others are not aware of the impending violence. Within a half-awake (hypnotic), reverie dream state he releases the repressed rage and experiences the violence as if it were real.

This experience is a "therapeutic abreaction." By reliving it through fantasy he does not need to carry it out in reality. However, such abreactions are usually initiated in psychotherapy with a nurturing therapist present. In this case his imagined "mother" takes that role. "She" would not let the enactment become real.

Adventures in Human Understanding

With the rage expressed and exhausted, guilt takes its place. He regresses again to childhood seeking the forgiveness and nurturance of his fantasied mother-therapist. She not only breaches the chasm between fantasy and reality in his understanding, but she takes him on further trips to understand the sources of anger in his persecutors.

Seeing that they, too, were rejected and bullied, he identifies with them and can no longer regard them as enemies to be killed.

The feeling of guilt, however, impels a need for restitution, even though his killing was only in fantasy. His mother-therapist points out a possible solution.

With much courage, he initiates an act of goodness toward his most hated persecutor, thus winning the plaudits and respect of his classmates. In this way, Goodwin enacts the wisdom of a very respected American statesman, Abraham Lincoln. When asked near the end of the Civil War how he, Lincoln, would deal with his enemies, the President replied, "I intend to eliminate them by turning them into friends."

Part II

The Summer of Life

Chapter 6

The "Hero" and his "Sister"

"Mom, how come I don't have a sister?"

As the only child of two aging, but loving parents Gilbert never had to compete for their attention. But there was no raucous laughter of playing youngsters in that home. Other boys had a sister. Why couldn't he?

Ellen brushed the slightly graying hair back and looked at her son with a thoughtful gaze. How should she answer him?

"We always wanted a girl, Son. But one just didn't come. Now it's too late. You're our only child, and we'll always love you." She didn't mention the little one they lost who had never gotten born.

As a 10-year-old Gilbert was lonely. There were few families with children in the community. But he was very competent and achieved every goal to which he put his mind. His parents knew he would be successful.

The few friends at school were not close, so Gilbert had much time to read and imagine. In addition to books, he read the *Reader's Digest* with special interest in its stories of heroes who rescued people in danger. They were always successful, like that tale of the boy who saved his sister from drowning when she fell into a raging river.

As the story told it, after hearing her screams, the boy had plunged into the torrent, dived deep into a whirlpool eddy, located her lifeless body and, struggling against cross-currents, towed her to safety, where, with artificial resuscitation, she was revived. That young man was a hero and forever honored in his community. Gilbert wished that he, too, could be a hero.

Adventures in Human Understanding

Of course, there was the swimming pool, the one center of recreation for teenagers in this small town. It was fun to lie on the warm concrete, watch the girls parade by in their skimpy swimsuits and let one's imagination go.

Somewhat smaller than the other boys, Gilbert nevertheless was a good swimmer, secured his junior and senior Red Cross life-saving badges, and competed at backstroke on the swimming team.

Now, armed with a bright, shiny Bachelor's degree (high honors) he was a young teacher in a rural high school. Times were hard, and he received the job because of his ability in music. For the modest salary offered, the school board couldn't find anybody else who agreed to teach algebra, geometry, business arithmetic, general science, physics, direct band, orchestra and coach debate. But Gilbert never doubted his competence. He expected to succeed.

On accepting the teaching assignment there he thought many of the farm kids rather dumb. Against his better judgment he had given a passing grade of "D" in Algebra to Roscoe, the football team's burly fullback.

Now it was June. School was out. There would be no more pay checks until September. He had to get a summer job. Bouncing planks behind the ripsaw of a lumber mill in a small forest community was the only one available.

It was Friday, 6:00 p.m., closing time at the Halleck and Howard lumber mill in Cascade. Gilbert was tired, very tired. Heaving 12-foot 2 × 10-inch planks up onto the adjacent lumber dolly as they emerged from the ripsaw was exhausting, especially when you had to keep it up for nine hours every day.

His partner at the mill was a big Swede called "Harry." Harry was the experienced lumberman who decided where the cuts would be made—and also the one who fed the logs into the ripsaw. Gilbert had always admired him and especially envied his broad chest and immense biceps. When Gilbert couldn't quite hoist that last big board to the top of the stack, Harry would laugh uproariously, take pity on "the kid," turn off the rotating saw blade, and bale him out.

With a sigh of relief Gilbert heard the siren scream, signaling the end of the shift. He dragged himself to the parking lot. Key in slot, the rusty old two-door Dodge sedan slowly chugged to life. Maybe he would feel better after a cool swim. The only place was a swimming hole in the Cascade river five miles away, where the locals, and especially the tired lumbermen, could take a dip after work. Gilbert headed there.

As he approached the stream he saw a small crowd, including a few fellow-workers from the mill, clustered about a body. Everybody seemed excited. A 15-year-old girl had jumped in over her head, and nobody had noticed until it was too late. Confusion reigned. There were shouts of, "Who found her?" "Why doesn't somebody help?" "Call a doctor." "How about the sheriff?"

Gilbert knew exactly what to do, administer resuscitation without delay. Suddenly, he became the expert. With masterful confidence he swung into action.

"Get back, everybody. Give her breathing room. Her head must be lower than her feet. Over there, where that slope is. Set her face down. Put something under her mouth and nose, so she doesn't swallow any sand."

A grizzled old logger pulled out a red bandanna handkerchief and stuffed it under her head.

Gilbert straddled the inert form and began the method he had learnt as a teenager from Peter Kim, the lifeguard at his hometown pool. Pushing down on her back, he repeated quietly to himself with each stroke, "Out goes the bad air; in comes the good. Out goes the bad air; in comes the good."

The crowd watched in silence, broken occasionally with a "When's she gonna start breathing?"

"Out goes the bad air; in comes the good. Out goes the bad air; in comes the good."

Gilbert pumped away vigorously flexing his thin biceps, perhaps somewhat strengthened by his month at the mill. Gone were the

Adventures in Human Understanding

feelings of fatigue; gone the thoughts of being a hero. Absent were any sexual feelings, which could have been aroused by the well-built figure of this girl. Complete concentration and only one idea governed his mind.

"Out goes the bad air; in comes the good. Out goes the bad air, in comes the good."

He recalled an instruction in the life-saving manual. "Somebody get a blanket to put over her." Two teenagers rushed to their cars, returning with a dirty brown blanket. Gilbert missed only one stroke while they were placing it over her.

Ten minutes passed, fifteen, twenty. Once, there was a gurgle, as some water came running out of her mouth. Everybody, including Gilbert, perked up. A good sign? Nothing came of it. A few of the older people in the crowd began shaking their heads. One woman had lost a son through drowning. Now memories of him, long suppressed, came to the fore. She began crying softly. Her gray-haired husband put his arm around her. Nobody noticed, least of all Gilbert. He was too busy.

"Out goes the bad air; in comes the good. Out goes the bad air, in comes the good."

Gilbert was tiring. Despondent thoughts hammered at the door of awareness. His arms were stiff, almost frozen with fatigue. But he forced the pain out of his mind. "She had to start breathing, she just had to." Everybody there was praying the same.

Exhausted, he paused a moment, took a deep breath, and stretched his arms outward. Then back to his job, his commitment, his duty.

"Out goes the bad air; in comes the good. Out goes the bad air; in comes the good." He was becoming discouraged and tried to push harder, but the effort was almost too much.

Now he noticed her as a person for the first time. Long blonde hair, beautiful shape, tanned back, orange one-piece bathing suit. Wouldn't she have made a wonderful sister, one like he had always hoped for? Perhaps if she lived he could get to know her, visit her family. Maybe she could be like a sister to him. Maybe.

"Out goes the bad air; in comes the good. Out goes the bad air; in comes the good."

Gilbert paused and looked up. "Listen everybody! It's too cold out here. We've got to get her to a warmer place. Has anybody got a truck?" Charlie Workman spoke up. "Mine's right over there, by that tree. I'll get it."

In another minute a mud-splattered, Model A Ford truck groaned to a halt near the unbreathing girl.

"Alright fellows. Put the blanket underneath and lift her in. Quick!"

A half-dozen willing hands picked up the crumpled form and shoved her onto the truck bed. Gilbert leaped upon the truck and again straddled the unmoving girl. He had only missed two cycles.

"Out goes the bad air; in comes the good. Out goes the bad air; in comes the good."

Charlie gunned the old truck. It took off with a roar, bumping over the rough forest road until it arrived at the brief, paved stretch near town. Seven minutes. That truck had never been pushed so fast.

By now Gilbert was getting desperate. It only took a few seconds to get her through the alley door. They laid her on the warm storeroom floor of Haveman's Mercantile—there being no hospital in town. Somebody called Sheriff Miller, a heavyset, powerfully built man. He rushed out of his office, stationed himself in front of the Mercantile's main door and, after being informed of what happened, addressed the gathering crowd in his usual commanding voice. "Move on. Move on. Everything's under control."

Gilbert's pushing movements slowed. "Out with the bad air. In—with—the—good. Out …" Realizing that her body was becoming stiff, he knew the battle was lost. Rigor mortis was setting in.

Adventures in Human Understanding

Tears flowed down his cheeks. Quickly he wiped them away with his hand. These tough loggers mustn't see him crying. A man doesn't cry. They would think him a weakling—which many of them at the mill probably thought already. He didn't notice there wasn't a dry eye among anybody there.

Slowly he slumped down and held his head in his arms. Then like a robot he stood up. He looked at nobody, and nobody looked at him. The entire room was filled with stillness. As he left no word was spoken, but at the door Harry was there, patted him on the shoulder, and said, "Tough going, Kid. You did all you could. Would you like a ride to get your car?" If it hadn't been unmanly, he could have hugged Harry at that moment.

Gilbert was totally devastated. He had failed at the most important job to which he had ever committed himself. He had used all of his knowledge, his skill, his energy—and the girl had died. He would be no hero. His "sister" was gone. He thought, "I wonder whether the men at the mill will think of me as a weakling, not competent, trying to be a hero when I just couldn't cut the mustard."

Monday when he reported for work, several of the fellows said, "Hi," and gave him a little touch as he went by. Two others joined Gilbert during lunch break. One offered to share a ham sandwich. Harry had informed the whole crew what happened last Friday.

The rest of the summer passed quickly. Somehow he seemed to relate more to these simple, rough loggers, most of whom had never gone to high school, and he felt different inside. He had experienced his first close contact with death—and had been defeated.

When school started in September Gilbert had almost forgotten his summer experience. He never mentioned it. However, the high school "kids" seemed to be brighter.

He thought, "They must have matured since last Spring. Maybe I should spend more time coaching Roscoe."

He did. To his surprise, Roscoe obtained a "C" in Geometry. Gilbert agreed it had been fully earned. Roscoe also ran for the winning touchdown that season against Hillsdale's constant rival, Walder—and became a "hero" to the community.

Thoughts of a Therapist: Analysis and Comment

Young Gilbert, a beginning schoolteacher (raised as an only child), has always wanted siblings, especially a sister. He reads stories of heroism, where, through super-human effort, the "hero" rescues a life. Slight of build, he dreams of the day when he, too, can dramatically rescue a drowning person through physical prowess.

Unlike many other young men, he has no great feelings of inferiority. He expects to meet his commitments and achieve his goals, having already demonstrated his competence in the field of academia. However, he does feel inferior physically, although he compensates by developing an insensitive attitude of superiority over others less gifted in scholarly pursuits.

Hard times and the need for summer income force him to accept a physically demanding job in a lumber mill. Through perseverance he performs his assigned tasks but can barely meet the demanding physical requirements. His good-natured partner, a strong, experienced lumberman, helps "the kid" out at times.

The chance for heroic accomplishment is offered when, at a community swimming hole in the river, an adolescent girl has been dragged out of the water. As an experienced swimmer with training in Red Cross life-saving methods, he is the only one there who knows what to do. He immediately takes charge.

With supreme confidence, he administers artificial resuscitation. He fantasizes himself as saving the girl's life, becoming a "hero," and acquiring "a sister."

Unfortunately, she has been underwater too long. He fails. With shaken confidence and unrealistic feelings of superiority gone, he must recognize he is only human.

Adventures in Human Understanding

Returning to work with humility, he finds the rough lumber workers appreciate his "heroic efforts" to save the girl. He senses a new respect from them. With greater understanding and compassionate feelings toward students, he resumes his teaching position the following September.

Chapter 7

The Novel

She was standing on the front porch, shouting a little louder than usual, "Joseph, have you got your raincoat?"

"I won't need it today, Mom."

"Oh yes, you will. I just heard the weatherman predicting rain storms this afternoon."

"Oh—kay," muttered Joseph, resentfully turning off the car key and returning to pick up his raincoat. After watching him drive off, his mother returned to the kitchen telephone.

"You still there, Margaret? That boy is so forgetful. Most of the time he does what he's supposed to, but occasionally he shows a stubborn streak—got it from his Dad. Now he has the crazy idea of making a train trip through Europe. I told him he should wait, then he and Mercedes could go together on their honeymoon."

"She's such a nice girl," volunteered Margaret.

"Yup!" replied Joseph's mother. "That girl's got a good head on her. She'll keep him in line, and I won't have to keep reminding him all the time."

Mom often talked to her best friend, Margaret, after Joseph left for work each morning. Later, she would muse to herself while washing the dishes: "Wouldn't it be nice if he would return to the seminary and complete his Doctor of Divinity degree? He could be ordained by the Church." She could almost see that sign in front of it: "Oaksdale First Methodist Church, Rev. Joseph Witherspoon, Pastor." The present minister was getting old. Folks said he would retire soon. Joseph and Mercedes could be married and then move into the parsonage, only two blocks down the street.

Adventures in Human Understanding

She had mentioned to Dick, her husband, how nice it would be to have them so close. They could visit their grandchildren every day. Dick agreed—but seemed somewhat hesitant.

Joseph had held a job as Counselor at a local employment service for three years, and he was good at it. However, life in the Witherspoon household was humdrum and uneventful until Joseph suddenly informed his mother he wanted a vacation and had signed up for this European tour. Being pushed for a reason, he had merely said, "I just want a little excitement before settling down."

This made no sense to Mom, but she realized that when he got in one of his "stubborn streaks" there was no use arguing with him. She also knew that in time he would feel guilty and come around to her way of thinking.

Joseph was regarded in the community as a reliable, but rather dull fellow. Solid, conscientious—never missed a day at the office. He seemed reconciled to bachelorhood, and lived at home. Most girls found him uninteresting. There was only Mercedes, his childhood sweetheart, with whom he occasionally went to the movies.

Five years earlier, at his mother's request, he had enrolled in a theological seminary, but after two semesters dropped out, entered graduate school, and completed a Master's degree in social work at the State University. Somewhat reconciled that at least he was in a helping profession, Mom had decided to postpone pushing for the Doctor of Divinity degree. There would be time later.

As an undergraduate Joseph had been attracted to romantic literature and had secret hopes of being a writer. In fact, he had been quietly working on a novel with visions of making the *New York Times* bestseller list, but had struggled for several weeks now to develop a satisfactory ending to its plot.

At State College, on the other side of Missouri, Madonna Heathcott taught English composition and literature. A tall, dark-haired, vivacious young woman with a sparkle in her eyes, she enjoyed making her students laugh when describing risqué tales of the Renaissance. While most women instructors were rather dowdy, Madonna appeared in outfits that were both brilliant-colored and daring. Dean Mathilda Grossmeyer, the gray-haired matriarch of the College, didn't quite approve of her. But what can you do when Madonna attracted enthusiastic enrollments in all her classes?

There were few unmarried men in their thirties at the school. But lacking any available alternative, she had become engaged to marry Kurt, the physics professor. Unbeknownst to him, however, she had planned to treat herself to a "fling" this summer. She would take a trip through Europe on the Orient Express before returning for the marriage. Kurt was not very supportive when she informed him of her decision.

"Listen, Madonna, what's this trip all about? I can't have you traipsing around overseas. We're engaged and supposed to get married. If you're going to be my wife, you'll have to straighten up and meet your obligations. I'd never permit my lab assistant to be so lackadaisical."

"Kurt, we're not married yet, and you can't push me around," announced Madonna.

Kurt was the best teacher in the college. He knew it and prided himself in spending much time preparing his lectures. Glowering, he retreated to his office.

Sometimes Madonna would bristle when he tried to control her behavior or personal views. She had determined to be her own person. However, after each brief quarrel she and Kurt usually reconciled and resumed their up-and-down relationship—which, of course, was aimed at marriage.

Madonna had been raised in a middle-class home where her mother was affectionate but not strong. Her father was a handsome man, rather dashing, admired by women, who made his living as a wholesale representative for a machine-products firm. This position required that he travel much of the time.

As a child she had worshipped him, and he returned her affection. In the family she was known as "Daddy's little girl." However, when she was thirteen he left the family after developing an affair with another woman, whom he had met on a business trip. His abandonment devastated Madonna. She felt that men could not be trusted. They would leave you. This conviction was reinforced by a few affairs she had in college with boyfriends. She had slept once with each, only to find that afterward they had no further interest in her. Accordingly, when she felt attracted toward a man she would withdraw into a passive neutrality that hid her underlying needs for warmth, affection, and closeness. She could seem to be energized in a non-emotional conversation, making her date feel important, even though she was not attracted to him. Several such relationships had come and gone.

Prospects of marriage dimmed until she began teaching at the same college as Kurt and decided he would make an acceptable husband. At least they did have their academic careers in the same institution. He would not be chasing other women and probably would never abandon her. She could feel safe with Kurt. However, there was always something missing. She just wasn't sure. This would be her last "fling" before getting married and settling down.

When Madonna opened the exterior compartment door of the train in Budapest she found she would be sharing it with a mild, neatly-appearing young fellow. Her first misgivings about being alone with this man were resolved when he was very courteous and lifted her bags to the overhead rack.

Madonna looked him over without appearing to do so. Well-dressed, dark suit, clean-cut features, blond, neatly-combed hair, tall, athletic build. He reminded her of somebody, but she couldn't decide just whom.

"Hm."

He seemed rather shy. Nothing much was said between them as the train slowly wound around the many curves in the track between Budapest and Vienna.

The Novel

Realizing that if there were to be any communication she would have to initiate it, Madonna inquired cautiously about his home, occupation and why he was taking this trip.

Although responding slowly at first, Joseph's interest began to pick up. He noticed that she was not only pleasant, but also very pretty. Her dark eyes looked at him as if he were "somebody." Women seldom showed any interest in him, and this obviously intelligent girl attracted him, especially when he found she taught English composition and literature in a college. With some misgivings he volunteered, "I'm writing a novel. Been working on it for two years, and think I have it almost finished."

Madonna, seeing this as a possible opening for conversation, responded with, "That sounds interesting. I'd like to hear more about it. Do you have a copy with you?"

"Well, yes. I try to write a little more each day, and I'm working now on the last chapter. It's just a hobby, you know. But it's something which none of my family ever did. Would you like to see it?"

Reaching into his briefcase, Joseph removed a dog-eared and obviously much thumbed sheaf of paper, most of which had been typewritten, but with a few more recent pages scribbled in pencil.

"That's what I've written since starting this trip," he explained.

Madonna took the manuscript and began skimming it. The story was about a dull set of experiences between a young man, "John," and "Mary," whose on-and-off relationship meandered aimlessly through church picnics, car breakdowns, an encounter with a snarling dog, arguments with family members, etc. It was very clear to her that this "novel" would never fly before a book publisher's editor. Not only was the story dull and uninspiring, but it was filled with platitudes and repetitions. It portrayed "John" and "Mary" as having been engaged for many years. Both families expected they would soon marry. John wanted to go somewhere, do something different, and not simply become another long-term resident in "Plentywood, Missouri." It was obvious, however, that "John" would always be a solid citizen, voting, upholding the law and perhaps running for the school board.

Adventures in Human Understanding

She recognized "John" was much like Joseph himself. But "Mary" was a vague individual. Joseph could not seem to develop a girl of substance or a personality for "Mary." To Madonna, she appeared as simply a stick figure, serving as a foil for "John's" interminable efforts to understand himself and establish self-determined goals. At times there flashed through the John character a glimmer of something that caused Madonna to continue reading with a new interest, especially when Joseph introduced into the plot an "attractive party girl," Genevieve.

Madonna increasingly realized that the entire novel was a portrayal of all that represented Joseph's past, present and plans for the future. What she saw did not inspire her. However, she also recognized that this was Joseph's creation, and he wanted her approval. Madonna tried offering some suggestions cautiously. She didn't want to offend him.

"That sentence where John warns Mary to beware of the snarling dog is written quite clearly, but if you put an exclamation mark after 'Look out' the punctuation would be more correct, and the sentence would have more power."

Joseph was impressed. "That's right. Thanks for the suggestion." He vigorously penned-in the correction and took another look at her. "I guess to teach English in college you have to be good in grammar and punctuation."

She continued making "suggestions." Soon she and Joseph were communicating and interacting, but in a way which was very safe for each. Clickety click, clickety click, clickety click. Many hours, many miles were spent as the train's engine plodded through rolling hills, passing through little towns, whose names were hard to pronounce. The reading of Joseph's manuscript encompassed more miles of dull, uninteresting fiction, as Madonna hoped to stimulate Joseph's personal interest in her.

The first break in this boring routine occurred when they reached Vienna. A two-day break in the scheduled "tour" was permitted. Although the tour company provided separate rooms for each traveler at the Queen Elizabeth hotel, Joseph found a few other

The Novel

ideas entering his mind as he was going to sleep. He did not dare act on them.

The next morning their tour guide suggested, "Why don't you take a bus around the city and then visit the Prater? It's a world-famous amusement park, you know."

"That sounds interesting," remarked Madonna, and Joseph agreed. Although they did not talk much, there was something very comforting sitting together. Madonna would ask his reactions to a number of the famous places they passed—city parks, Freud's home, Strauss's and many others.

The next day at the Prater, Madonna, like an excited child, insisted, "Let's go up on the big Ferris wheel. My Dad used to take me to one in Kansas City."

This one indeed looked high to Joseph. "You think it's safe?"

"Come on. It's going to be real fun," reacted Madonna.

At first Joseph was dubious. But soon he, too, was enjoying the excitement—especially when at the top Madonna would grab his hand and hold on.

"Wow!" she screamed, peals of laughter sweeping over her pretty face.

Joseph wanted to reach over and kiss her, but he didn't dare. However, it made him feel important, as if he were protecting her. After a lunch of beer and wurst they returned to the hotel.

The last night the tour provided tickets to the opera. The performance excited the imagination of both, and Madonna cried when Carmen died. This shocked Joseph. One shouldn't cry in public. Still, with his eyes almost moist, he patted her shoulder, to which she made no objection. The two days had been filled with more excitement and "adventure" than either had ever experienced. They talked constantly.

Adventures in Human Understanding

From Vienna to Zurich both were less rigid. Frequently they shared a laugh. However, their ingrained pattern of insecurities continued. Even the beautiful scenery of the Austrian Alps at Innsbruck did not excite them. Joseph seemed once more completely absorbed within himself.

Madonna, deciding he must be bored with her, picked up the English language edition of *Time*, having acquired it at a little bookstore in Vienna, and resumed reading. The train approached Zurich. Joseph returned to writing on his novel. There was little change in its theme. The young man, "John," was caught up in a restrictive environment, a dutiful son to a controlling mother. He would marry "Mary." They would settle down to a comfortable, small-town existence. "John's" feelings that he was not worthy of a woman's attraction and love continued, as represented in many incidents throughout the manuscript.

Madonna, however, had become increasingly attracted to Joseph. He was a handsome man, sincere appearing, courteous and attentive to her in a non-erotic manner. In many ways he was like her father, whom she still admired and loved in spite of his infidelity to her mother. However, this, in itself, reminded her of the faithlessness of men. Reinforced by her few experiences in college, it kept her behavior toward Joseph "proper." This proper behavior in turn reinforced Joseph's conviction that he could not really be loved by a woman. He remained tongue-tied, his passivity concealing a whirlwind of inner reflection.

At the urging of a friend in college he had once visited a prostitute. The experience was pleasurable. It was also disgusting and had turned him away from women. In his perception there were two kinds of women: Those who wouldn't be interested in him, because he was "unattractive," and those who were cheap, vulgar and disgusting.

A day before the Orient Express trip would end in Paris he closed his manuscript, sighed and spoke to her. "Well, I've finished it now. Got all the problems solved. Would you like to hear how the story finally came out?"

"I'd be very interested in the ending. Love to have you read it to me," she replied with misgivings. Joseph began reading. In the novel all the minor obstacles had been overcome. The main character, "John," deciding he should not be distracted from his original goals, had broken off his interest in "Genevieve." He would ask Mary formally to marry him. The novel was finished. With a satisfied smile Joseph completed reading the last chapter to her, then filed it away in his briefcase.

Madonna slumped dejectedly back in her seat. "I guess you must feel relief now that it's finished?"

It was obvious that Joseph would never achieve independence from his background. She thought, "I might as well return to State College and marry Kurt." Joseph was handsome and stable. She knew he would make a good husband, one on whom you could depend. He would never abandon her as her father and boyfriends had, but he would be boring.

She sighed sadly to herself, "I suppose he'll always be tied to his mother."

It was almost dark when they left Zurich on the overnight trip to Paris. The other occupants of their cabin had left at Zurich. The express barreled through the hills and valleys of Switzerland. A drizzling rain outside the cabin window only added to Madonna's feeling of hopelessness. With the compartment to themselves and privacy for the night, they each had a full seat on which to recline. Extracting a blanket from overhead, Madonna decided to lie down. Soon she was fast asleep.

The train raced through Belgium toward Paris. Except for the normal train noise, all was quiet. Only one dim light illuminated the compartment.

Joseph, however, was wide awake. He felt more alert than ever before. His brain, normally slow, was racing like the powerful train in which they were riding. The clickety click of the train wheels eliminated all distractions and stimulated his mental and emotional processes.

Adventures in Human Understanding

Thoughts, more thoughts, ideas, wishes, hopes, fantasies poured out in abundance, as if a horn of plenty were divesting its fruits in all directions. It seemed as if his whole life was spread out before him—like a vast multi-colored tapestry. His early childhood, his affectionate but controlling parents, his struggles in grade school, his shyness with girls, the experience with the prostitute, his year at the divinity school, the social-work graduate school.

It was much later at night when Joseph reached a decision. He must revise his novel. Scribbling furiously for almost an hour, he rewrote the plot and then returned the manuscript to his briefcase. Exhausted, he retrieved a blanket, lay down, and he too was soon in a dreamless sleep.

On and on the train roared as the two young people slumbered, oblivious of the grinding wheels and the occasional horn, as the engine forged its way through the darkness of the Belgian countryside.

Suddenly there was a jerk in the car. Startled, Madonna opened her eyes and for a moment wondered just where she was. Oh yes, she and Joseph were bound on a train—to nowhere. She had placed such hopes on the possibility that Joseph could be changed and would make a good husband. He had so many of the traits to which she was attracted. She truly admired him, but the ending of his novel told her that any further relationship was an invitation into a blind alley.

Was it Joseph that was a failure? Could she have done something different? She thought about this, her last "fling," which had turned into a dud. Why could she have possibly believed it all would end differently?

Compulsively her meanderings kept turning toward Joseph, his personality, the cues to his behavior which she had picked up from his novel, and from her woman's intuition. Was he really this stick, hopelessly entrapped in his restricting world? Or could he break out of it? Did he really want to? Was it possible that underneath that shyness there were some smoldering coals? Had she, because of her own fears and her "proper" behavior, turned him off?

Maybe there was something that she had not yet discovered. The more she gazed at him resting there, the more desirable he looked.

Finally, a daring impulse crossed her mind. She dismissed it, but the thought kept returning again and again until it almost became an obsession. She had to know, what was he really like? And she had to know now before they reached Paris.

Could she dare? Maybe. What had she to lose? Obsession turned to conviction. No one could look in the window. There were no more stops. The conductor had paid his last visit for the night. Their privacy was complete.

Noiselessly removing her clothes, she stood up, a modern Aphrodite in alabaster and pink. Moving over to his side, she pulled back his blanket. Sitting astride him she unzipped his pants.

Joseph awoke suddenly, as if he had been precipitated into the here-and-now by the explosion of a nuclear bomb. Startled, it took him several seconds to understand this "happening."

He mumbled, "Uh! Uh! What! Oh!" as his physiology rose to the occasion.

Feeling as if he had been suddenly transported to paradise, and with his head in a whirl, he desperately grabbed the engine of his emotions and tried to hang on. Clearly there was no stopping this fast express until it reached its destination.

The thunder and lightnings of their passions built and built as two bodies, two selves, strove toward a fusion of being. And then—and then—suddenly heavenly reservoirs burst open. A deluge of ecstasy inundated the famished lands, flooding them with a common sea of life-sustaining oneness—which, like the rites of spring, had for centuries portended a new flowering.

Rapidly as it had started, it was over. Movement and breathing almost stopped. Peace prevailed over their world, broken but slightly by the clickety click of the train's wheels, carrying them to a common destiny. They lay beside each other, slowly unwinding,

Adventures in Human Understanding

and gazing at each other with a new light in their eyes. No words were spoken. Each one knew. Yes, each one knew. But what was it that each one knew?

Silently Madonna returned to her side of the compartment, donned her clothing, lay down, and faded into a reverie. She had proved that Joseph was not impotent, not too shy to be an erotic partner. He was lovable. He could be a man. She felt good about that. And she knew that any woman who received his commitment would be his lifelong partner. He was everything she wanted, but he had said nothing—just turned over on his side and appeared to be sleeping.

Maybe after he returned home he would remember these few moments of passion. Maybe he would know that there was a woman who truly loved him, one who was not cheap or tawdry, one who had presented him with the gift of her total self. Perhaps he would respect her. Perhaps not.

But was it important? He had already told her his life decision. "John" would marry "Mary," and Joseph would return home to Mercedes. Like all other men, he would leave her.

She could find no way to surmount this last great obstacle. She had gambled, and she had lost, even as Carmen in the opera had lost. But what had she really lost? She truly loved him, and so she had lost no self-respect. It was not like those boys in college. She could survive, and Kurt would be waiting for her. The great cloud of sadness again shadowed her thoughts until healing slumber enveloped her.

Joseph lay quietly on the seat staring at the ceiling. Glancing from time to time at the sleeping Madonna, he would shake his head, make motions in the air, as if he were trying to solve some complex problem.

In a few electrifying moments this beautiful woman had proved to him that he was an attractive, exciting and lovable man. He could no longer doubt that. His feelings of inferiority from childhood had been smashed as if run over by the engine of her passion. And his own had been roused to an equal intensity.

If Mom knew of this episode she would strongly disapprove. To hell with Mother. He loved her, but he would no longer let her rule his life. He would do what he wanted to do, what he needed to do, whether she approved or not.

One last sticking point came to mind. Was Madonna a harlot, who climbed in bed with every man? Was she like that prostitute? He remembered the experience with that woman, long stringy hair, heavily rouged cheeks, dark circles under her eyes painted blue, short pants, leather leggings. She had treated him like a little kid. "Get it on, honey. Hurry up."

Afterward, she had simply grabbed the 50-dollar bill and disappeared down the stairs of the dingy little hotel. He recalled vividly how cheap and put-down he felt. No! Absolutely not! This intimacy was totally different. Nothing in this experience resembled that with the prostitute. Madonna was simply not the same kind of woman. She really loved him, gave him the most desirable gift of her self, and left him feeling like a man, grown-up, mature. More than anything else he wanted to share his life with her.

Madonna had listened patiently to his "novel," which he realized now was a feeble portrayal of his own meaningless life. It was a lousy story. No publisher would ever take it. But she, in her gentle way, had not criticized; she had not ridiculed; she had shown him the utmost respect. Respect and love, that's what he had always really wanted.

He knew now the novel was not worth keeping, but he must show it to her one more time. He would ask her to judge it and himself now. He must convey to her the last revised chapter.

With considerable misgivings and shaking hand he extracted it from the briefcase, awakened her, and said, "Madonna, last night, when you slept I concluded that I had not written the ending of my novel as I really feel. Then I didn't believe that I would have the courage to show it to you again. But you gave me the strength to do so. Would you mind listening to the revision of that last chapter?"

Adventures in Human Understanding

Madonna thought, "Why now, after it is all over? Why would he still want my reactions to the novel?" Puzzled, and anticipating another round of dull interactions between "John" and "Mary," she settled down while Joseph began reading in a much firmer voice than usual.

"John realized that this was his life's decision. He had made many wrong ones before. But now there was no turning back. He either returned to that small town, settled down with Mercedes—I mean Mary—whom he had never really loved, or embarked on the most exciting adventure of his life with that wonderful woman whom he had just discovered, Genevieve. He knew now who was his real sweetheart, who would give him the deep love and understanding he always wanted. Would she consent to share this adventure with him? He still had some lingering doubts about his ability to please her, to keep her interested in him, but he knew that he could never leave her, that if she said, 'Yes,' they would be together until the end of their days.

"He would give her everything he had to give, everything in his life, his being, his existence. He would be a child no longer. He had not been fair with 'Mary,' letting her think he was in love with her. He would pen a kindly goodbye. He must now be true to himself and be fair with everyone. He had not been fair with 'Genevieve.' Under a feeling that he was unworthy and unlovable, he had concealed from her his real self. He must tell her now, before it was too late. She had to know his true feelings and who he really was."

Laying the manuscript aside, taking Madonna's hands into his, and looking deeply into her eyes Joseph softly said, "I want to read you a little poem. I thought it was 'John' who had written it to 'Genevieve.' I realize now that it was me writing to you."

> Tell me, My Dearest.
> Now that I have found thee,
> That the light which in thine eyes
> Shines on my gaze, with warmth
> Like the sun.
> 'Twill always grace my being
> With a closeness unto thee.
> I dare not ask for more.

But pledge you all I have
The realness of my self
To be your chosen spouse.
If you will spend your days
As my beloved wife.

"These words came from me, and I wrote them for you, Madonna. But I dared not speak them except through the lips of an imaginary 'John,' a fumbling child, who never did find himself. For several days now, your presence has been always on my mind. But somehow, I had to know, to prove to myself, that I need be a boy no longer. That I am a man. This man wants to spend the rest of his life with you."

No words were spoken. Her smile, the loving touch and the arms about his shoulders gave eloquently her answer.

The glow in the eastern sky began brightening. The clouds were lifting. Soon all darkness disappeared, and the train burst out into the morning sunshine of a new day.

Thoughts of a Therapist: Analysis and Comment

Many people find life partners who are not "right" for them, others are more successful. The average marriage today lasts less than ten years. Courting and mating rituals are challenging, especially if they come later in life than normal. Joseph and Madonna are two just such people.

Opposing a controlling mother, to whom he had been obedient all of his life, is an ordeal for Joseph. He desperately wants to become independent. He fantasizes a happy married life and tries to write a romance novel but has neither the experience nor imagination to make it realistic. Discouraged and confused, he will try, before settling down, a last adventure in the hope that somehow a new experience will happen.

Madonna has already matured out of childhood, but the college world offers few marriageable males in her age range. With no other options she must settle for a mediocre relationship, even if she has to battle to keep from being dominated. She, too, will try one last "fling."

By chance the two parties meet in a train compartment and warily contact each other. Madonna is attracted to Joseph but is very suspicious of all men because "they will be unfaithful in marriage and will abandon you," as did her father.

Joseph has little experience with women and divides them into two classes: Respectable, attractive girls who are not interested in him, and cheap "prostitutes." Their respective immaturities and past experiences keep their interaction on polite terms—although after Vienna the ice is somewhat broken.

In the meantime there are many covert communications going on between them. He is courteous. To her, his shyness is attractive. She looks at him "as if he were somebody." He is not accustomed to such attention. She wants to "listen" to his novel and is respectfully helpful. He had expected criticism. In his novel-character "Genevieve," Joseph hints at a spark within.

Atop the Ferris wheel Madonna clings to him—stimulating his masculine need to take care of others—already present in his human service careers, social work, counseling.

Madonna recognizes him as probably a good husband, loyal, one who won't run around or abandon her. However, she has one question: Is he a man or a boy? Can he respond appropriately to a mature sexual love? (Unconsciously, could they have children?)

Joseph is confused by her seeming interest in him, but he wonders if she will be promiscuous. Each needs an answer to their unverbalized questions.

Madonna, the stronger of the two, decides to put hers to test. She gambles and satisfies her question. But will he now respect her?

Joseph has already answered his question. He writes his response into the "novel," which he dares to read to her. The two "rescue" each other from unsatisfying marriages.

Joseph first signaled a spark of independence from his mother when he left the theological seminary. Had he remained he would have met his mother's dream, but probably been a mediocre pastor. Lacking experience in living, his ministry would have consisted of boring sermons, platitudes and enjoining his parishioners to "do good."

Madonna escaped an unhappy and conflictual marriage, probably headed for divorce unless she were to surrender to Kurt's bullying.

If Kurt is unable to find some younger woman who seeks a dominating father figure, he may retreat into a rigid bachelorhood. Life satisfactions would be based on his lecturing skill at teaching the laws of non-living matter.

Madonna will strengthen Joseph's independence. She will not accept his mother residing nearby, trying to control the rearing of their children.

Mom's fate if she does not develop more insight and flexibility? An unhappy old woman, critical of her daughter-in-law, trying to split up the marriage, and complaining to her friends.

Chapter 8

The Therapist

"God-damn-it," shouted George Henderson, "the toast is burned again. Can't you ever learn to make decent toast?" Mabel, not one to retreat from a fight, struck back, "If we could afford a new toaster instead of that cheap old thing you bought me 20 years ago, you'd have good toast." Then, not willing to abandon the fray yet, she inserted the stiletto a little deeper.

"Maybe if you were more of a man, like my brother Henry, you'd bring home enough money, so we could buy a new one." A below-the-belt hit like this could always be counted on to spark an explosion.

George was one of the baby-boom generation, too old to be fooling around, not old enough to have established respect as a senior. His baggy pants and receding hairline did not present an impressive appearance. Perhaps that was why he hadn't received the promotion, which he felt was deserved.

Henry had graduated from the University with a degree in business administration. A year ago, he had applied for a job at the construction firm where George worked.

George, who had a junior college degree, was a supervisor in the firm's Personnel Department. He had sponsored Henry's application and skippered it through successfully. Shortly afterward, Henry was promoted to Assistant Manager in charge of production. Mabel knew she had to only mention Henry's name to blow George's fuse.

"Shit! You women are all alike, bitch, complain and nag." George threw down his newspaper and stomped out of the room.

Mabel slumped her 215 pounds into a chair, forked another sausage and began wolfing it down. When eating, she resembled a

Adventures in Human Understanding

ravenous leopard with a newly downed gazelle. This, in addition to snacking throughout the day, had been a source of both comfort and grief. Temporarily satisfied, she could embark on the daily chores with her usual compulsive restlessness. But then the bathroom scale would soar another two pounds. Depression would once more descend upon her.

A half-hour later George stormed into his office, still pissed-off at Mabel's remark about Henry and muttering to himself, "I've worked my ass off providing a good living for her. No appreciation, just nag, nag, nag."

Caroline, typing up a report, leaned over to the new clerk, "Here comes Old Grouch. Don't say a word."

George glared at her. "Where's that file on the new Sales Manager? Did you lose it again?"

Caroline, a slender 118-pound good-looker with long wavy blonde hair, sat a little straighter in her desk chair. In this office one must appear to be working hard, even when there wasn't much to do. George could become quite angry at any little signs of inefficiency. Caroline, who had learned to survive some 12 years of George's tirades, picked up a folder and handed it to him.

"Here it is, Boss, all ready for your decision." George calmed down. At least there was one woman who appreciated his intelligence.

At home, Mabel had finished the dishes and cleaned up the kitchen. She picked up the newspaper from the floor and began searching for "Dear Abby." Every day after George left she read it studiously. Occasionally she glanced at the six-by-eight, rosewood framed photo on the mantel that displayed an attractive, slim young woman in a wedding dress, standing beside a stiff-looking, thirtyish man. There were three-striped badges on each sleeve of his Vietnam War uniform. A number of ribbons were pinned on the young soldier's chest proclaiming that he had done a meritorious job as a platoon sergeant.

The Therapist

Mabel's feeling of bitterness returned, occasionally broken by a single tear, quickly wiped off by a Kleenex. She still had satin-skin and rosy cheeks, belying the almost half century since a white-clad doctor had announced to her unenthusiastic mother, "A healthy baby girl." However, the favorable impression her features should have evoked was diminished by the constant scowl that engulfed them.

When they were first married Mabel would get up early, apply the necessary lipstick, and comb out her flowing light brown tresses. She wanted George to see her the way she looked that night at the Senior ball when he had cut in.

In those days that quick kiss and the hurried, "Bye, Honey," as he rushed out the door had assured he would remember her throughout the day, and never look twice at that new snip of a girl, Caroline, who had just been hired as the company secretary. Not that George was the roaming type, but you know how men are, and Mabel took no chances then. But now her stringy hair was prematurely tinged with gray, and the chore of combing it wasn't worth the bother.

The house was a large, two-story clapboard structure. The 45-year-old dwelling in a neighborhood that had seen its best days was badly in need of painting. The yard was rimmed by meant-to-be flower beds filled with weeds.

It was early September, and the tired old summer was expiring. A few leaves on the maple tree in the front yard were already turning russet. Mabel felt too worn out to do any more, so she just lay on the couch sadly reminiscing about the days back in the springtime of their life together.

They had stretched their finances, and borrowed to the limit to get this place. It was intended by now to be filled with the happy voices of little children. Mabel had become pregnant once, but three months later lost it, a little son. She had planned to name him "George, Jr." There were no more pregnancies, and in time they quit trying. Now they were saddled with a big debt and an old house much too large for two people. For Mabel, it was drudgery

Adventures in Human Understanding

to keep it clean and neat, especially when George never picked up anything. Sometimes a call to her sister, Emily, helped.

"Emily, just wondered what you were doing. George got mad at me again, complained of the breakfast, and stormed out. Why do men never care about the extra work they make for women?"

"You think you've got it bad, Mabel. You should be married to Doug. Last night he came in, roaring drunk, yelling at me, demanding sex. Is that what every man's got on his mind? I'd leave him if it weren't for the kids." And so it went for almost an hour, when Mabel, remembering a dental appointment, hung up.

It was about four o'clock when the phone rang. George's voice, "Wanted to let you know I have to work late tonight. Thought I'd get something to eat at The Club, maybe play a game or two with the boys just to get the pressure down. I'll be home by eleven." This happened once or twice a week.

"Humph," snorted Mabel to herself. "I know that's what he's really doing. Not stepping out on me. But sometimes I wonder about that sleek-looking blonde secretary, Caroline. She keeps her job by flattering him. He'll probably still be in his foul mood when he gets home. Might as well go to bed and read."

At The Club the usual group of poker players were absent from their corner table. So George cozied up to the bar beside Wayne, an old high-school buddy. George ordered a beer. Much talk about the election campaign and what the 49ers would do this year.

He and Wayne had made almost a ritual of reminiscing over a beer every so often. Wayne had been student-body president, and in George's eyes was a real smart guy. When things went wrong he could always count on Wayne for a sympathetic ear. This time, however, it was Wayne who suddenly interrupted the conversation.

"What gives these days with you and Mabel?"

"What do you mean, what gives?" growled George, belligerently.

"You know! You're always grumbling at each other. In fact, you two act like you hate each other—no love anymore."

"No love? Of course we love each other. Why do you think I've put up with her nagging for 19 years? You get married and stay married because you love your wife."

"Sure doesn't look that way to me. Why don't you two see a counselor or a therapist? Might help matters."

George exploded. "Me see a shrink! No deal. I'm not crazy just 'cause my wife is always bitching. Of course we love each other."

Wayne retreated into silence. Sullenly George finished his beer and, putting on his jacket, braved the driving rain outside to two blocks away where the car was parked. George talked a lot to himself. "See a psychiatrist? What does he think I am? Nuts?"

The storm was still raging with gusts and drenching sheets of rain when George slunk into his house at eleven-fifteen, completely soaked. "Had some trouble getting the car started. The carburetor must have gotten wet." Mabel said nothing. She was almost asleep in the middle of the big king-sized bed.

George, tossing his coat on the still warm living-room couch, shuffled downstairs to his study. Safely there, he didn't have to listen to Mabel's yakking. Too tired to undress, he kicked off his shoes and, pulling up the blanket on the makeshift couch, was soon asleep.

It was dark outside when he was startled by the sound of Mabel's voice shouting, "George, wake up! There's somebody trying to get in the house."

George, half-asleep, resentfully blinked his eyes open. The storm was still going full blast. But he could hear a banging outside near the porch "What time is it? Four-thirty? Too damned early. Maybe I'd better go take a look."

Adventures in Human Understanding

Climbing the stairs back up to the first floor was a real chore. "What the hell is going on," he wondered as he forced open the front door against the surging wind? He saw nothing there.

"Probably just some shingles flapping." Someday he'd climb up on the roof and replace them. Maybe he'd fall off and get killed. Mabel wouldn't care. She'd get that fifty-thousand dollars insurance. Then she'd be happy.

However, just as he was closing the door and looking forward to a warm bed, he noticed a black blob on the first step of the porch. It didn't move. Probably just a piece of drift wood blown there by the storm. He looked a little closer.

"Well I'll be damned! A dead cat. Must have been hanging to the tree branch. Got washed off when it bumped the porch. Tried to climb the stairs and couldn't make it past the first step before it died."

"What is it?" came Mabel's anxious voice from the back bedroom. "Nothing, just a dead cat, a little black one."

Mabel felt very annoyed. How come they had to have a dead cat washed up on their porch? "Well, throw it in the garbage and go to bed."

George headed for the garbage can on the back porch carrying the dead cat by one leg when he heard a slight "Meow" and felt a feeble movement. He really wasn't sure he'd heard anything, so he lifted the cat up to his ear. Sure enough, it was breathing, but barely so.

"Hey Mabel, this cat's still alive."

"Alive?" This posed a puzzling problem. "Well, we can't keep a cat. Lock it on the back porch. We'll turn it in to the pound tomorrow. Maybe someone will claim it."

George obeyed. Mabel settled back and tried to sleep. She kept tossing back and forth getting more and more awake. "Poor little kitten. At least it needed a better place to rest than the bare back porch."

Finally, still bothered, she got up and found a ragged blanket in the dust closet. Then, shivering her way to the back porch, she wadded the cloth into a little bed in the corner and placed the limp, motionless body of the kitten on it.

"Probably be dead in the morning, but what can I do? Too bad. It does look kinda cute."

George was up early the next morning. The city pound was on the other side of town. If he were to get to work on time he'd better start moving.

"Don't bother about breakfast. I've got the cat, and I'm leaving for the pound."

Mabel threw the covers back, "Hey! Wait a minute, George. Why don't we just keep it a few days? Put a notice in the paper. Probably the owner who lost it will call." Mabel's frustrated maternal instinct was stirring.

George left for the office and phoned in a short notice to the lost-and-found column of the *Hillsboro Daily Courier*. Nothing came of it. That weekend a conference was held. George thought the cat would be a nuisance. He wanted to take it immediately to the pound. But Mabel was adamant. "Suppose nobody claims it. Then they'll put it to sleep. Do we want that to happen?" George agreed it wouldn't be fair to the cat. So it stayed.

In a few days, with saucers of milk, morsels of food, and concerned care, the kitten brightened up. Within a week it was nosing around, exploring the whole house. George didn't take it kindly when he had to clean up a mess in the dining room.

"How can you blame a little kitten for just being natural," Mabel declared. That set George to thinking again.

Adventures in Human Understanding

"Mabel, I've got an idea. Why don't we buy one of those kitty-litter boxes you read about? You fill it with sand, and she can do her thing there. No more mess."

That sounded good to Mabel who was tired of cleaning up messes. She started to snipe, something about George's messes, thought better, bit her tongue, and shut up.

They couldn't keep calling her just "the cat," so the name "Elizabeth" was agreed upon—because George said she looked like a queen. Elizabeth, sometimes just "Lizzy," began her reign of the Henderson household.

George built a ledge on the kitchen window where she could crouch while watching the birds and squirrels in the backyard trees. At breakfast, he and Mabel would muse how cute she looked there. And each evening, when he got home, George wanted a complete rundown of what Lizzy had done that day.

"Well! She kept climbing on my lap and wanted to be petted. I could hardly get my work done."

George felt rather jealous. How come he didn't get to pet the cat more often? So, while watching the six o'clock newscast on NBC, he would invite Elizabeth to jump up on his lap, and somehow managed to combine stroking her with snorting at the political speeches.

One morning Elizabeth didn't climb up to her window perch. She looked sick. In great agitation Mabel dialed the office. "George, Lizzy's sick. She's coughing and gagging. We've got to get her to the vet."

"Thanks for calling. I'll take off right now."

After he rushed out of the office, Caroline observed, "Well, what's that all about? Never seen him move that fast before."

When Mabel heard George park in the driveway and run up the front steps she was waiting with Elizabeth wrapped in a blanket, the new expensive one with the fancy artwork.

"My God, Mabel! What's the matter with her? Is she going to die? I'll get us there as fast as I can."

The 1991 Plymouth Suburban sped down Walnut Street onto the Freeway and turned right at the off-ramp onto Broadway. Two blocks later they parked in front of a small brown building. The sign read, "Dr. Wilson's Cats on Broadway Hospital." Fortunately the policeman who patrolled that section of town was exchanging jokes with a couple of buddies over their usual morning coffee-break at Ruby's Café. The last thing George needed at that time was a speeding ticket.

Dr. Wilson quickly realized that George and Mabel were more "ill" than Elizabeth. After some reassurance, she explained to them, "It's only a hair ball which Elizabeth gets from licking her fur. That's her way of cleaning herself. Here's some medicine for it. When she acts this way let her lick this petroleum jelly. The hair ball will come out in her litter box, and you don't need to worry."

As they got in the car with their precious bundle, George impulsively reached over and gave Mabel a little peck on the cheek. Mabel just smiled. "Thanks for coming home so quickly." And George thought, "When it comes to Lizzy, Mabel and I are pretty good parents."

A new problem reared itself. Each morning when Elizabeth crawled out of her sleeping pad on the back porch, she wanted to get in bed with Mabel or George. She was always welcomed by each with "baby talk" and a great deal of stroking. She would spend a few minutes with Mabel, then scurry downstairs to snuggle with George. The difficulty needed a solution. It was resolved when they decided that maybe they could both share the king-sized bed in Mabel's room again. However, they still slept as far apart as possible.

Elizabeth kept repeating this unusual behavior, meowing and running back and forth from one side of the bed to the other. Each time she snuggled her head for a few minutes, first under Mabel's chin then under George's.

A better solution seemed to suggest itself. If they moved closer together, about one foot apart, Elizabeth could sleep between, and they could both pat her at the same time. Sometimes in a drowsy state the "patting" missed the cat and reached the other's shoulder.

Many changes now appeared in the household. George stopped working late. At breakfast the toast never got burned. George even remembered to put the toilet seat down. And Mabel found less clutter in the living room.

She smiled more often, and George enjoyed greeting her each morning with, "Hi, Dear." Her smile, which followed, reminded him of their first Coke-date 20 years ago.

When George stopped by her chair and rubbed her neck, Mabel also purred (like Elizabeth). Her hair was neatly combed more often, and either she forgot to nag, or George didn't notice it.

One evening the following October they were chatting together. Elizabeth was outside chasing Caesar, the pet squirrel who eagerly consumed the peanuts that were occasionally dropped in the crotch of the big maple. Suddenly there was a screeching of brakes and a loud cry. Overwhelmed by fear they both tried to rush out the front door at the same time.

It was Karl Peterson, their next-door neighbor, shouting and pointing. Karl was a widower, 72 years old. He lived alone ever since his wife had died five years ago. Mabel would occasionally take over a plateful of her prized cookies, and he in turn would often shovel the snow off their walks during winter.

"That red convertible jammed on his brakes, but when he saw what he had done to your cat, the son-of-a-bitch just high-tailed it onto the highway."

Many neighbors were looking out their doors now as George and Mabel rushed to the corner and picked up the inert form of Elizabeth.

"Oh my baby. My baby," wailed Mabel, cuddling the little crushed black ball, which was covered with blood. "For God's sake, call Dr. Wilson now. Maybe Lizzy's still alive."

George took one look and knew that Elizabeth was beyond rescue. He tried to hold the tears back. A man mustn't cry. But he could no longer refrain when his friends and neighbors clustered round, trying to say something reassuring.

With one arm carrying Elizabeth and the other around Mabel, he stumbled up the steps of their porch. The crushed form of Elizabeth was wrapped in a towel, and placed on the living room coffee table. Then the two of them sat, crying together and hugging each other.

It was an hour later when George stirred and said, "I guess we'll have to bury her."

Mabel wiped the tears away. "Why don't you dig a grave under the lilac bush in the back yard? Then we'll always have her close to us."

George looked thoughtful for a few moments. He didn't want to disappoint Mabel. Finally he remarked, "I'm sorry, Dear, but it's against the city ordinances to bury an animal within the city limits—and besides the neighbors would object. We'll take her to Dr. Wilson. She'll know what to do."

When George and Mabel brought in Elizabeth's body and told her the story of what had happened, Dr. Wilson cried with them. Ultimately professional competence came to the fore, and she said, "I'll take her body and dispose of it. It will be cremated."

The long winter finally wore itself out. Many evenings George and Mabel had sat together on the living room couch staring at the TV. Nothing interested them, not even *The Wheel of Fortune*—to which Mabel was addicted. After a long period of sitting it was usually Mabel who managed to start a conversation.

Adventures in Human Understanding

"Do you remember how Lizzy would roll on her back to welcome us back home after we'd been out? She sure was cute."

"Yeah! But she liked you better than me."

"How so?"

"Well, you know she would like having you rub her belly. I guess she didn't trust me. When I touched her there she would grab my fingers in her claws."

"I don't think she liked me any better. It was just that when she smelled the open can of tuna in the refrigerator she knew she could get me to give in and get her some if she begged long enough. You were more tough with her."

A half-smile came over George's face.

"Do you remember that time she brought you a gift, a dead sparrow?" The chuckle turned into a full-sized laugh. "I thought you'd never get over it."

"Well, it wasn't very nice of her, and I scolded her."

"Ha! You didn't think it changed her nature, did you?"

And so it would go on for some time. In many ways Elizabeth had showered affection on George and Mabel, and they had felt loved.

One evening, as spring approached, they were reading in the living room when unexpectedly Mabel turned to George and said, "I'd like to tell you about my early life. I don't think we ever talked about it."

This unusual overture surprised him, but putting down the newspaper, he leaned back in his easy chair and listened.

"Dad left us kids when I was very young. We were raised by Mother. She worked hard, but there was little affection. I always wanted to feel loved, but I wasn't. Guess when I married you I thought we'd make up for that. How was it with you?"

George was taken aback by such unaccustomed frankness. She had started this intimacy. He felt impelled now to share more of himself.

"My Dad was a mean bastard. He would come home and beat us kids with his razor strop. I often wanted to run away, but Mother seemed so helpless. I needed to protect her. Guess I was angry at her too. She never stood up to him or protected me." This was the first of a number of such "sharing talks." They began to discover how human the other was, and how they each had the same needs.

Winter was gone. It was the first year George didn't get the flu. He seemed to be more efficient at the office, and the boss gave him an unexpected raise. Mabel was planning how to seed the flower beds this year. George often found her humming to herself while she worked around the house. One day another of George's "ideas" emerged.

"We need to get out, Mabel. How about my reserving a table tomorrow night at the Elk's Club? They've got a new band, and they're serving crab legs. Can an old crab make a date with a young gal like you?" He laughed uproariously at his own joke.

When George came home that evening he found her rummaging through the closet. It was filled with many expensive dresses, bought years ago before they had splurged on the house. Most of them were several sizes too small. No matter how many Mabel tried to worm into, only a few were now possible. She decided that most were lost causes and gave them the next day to Good Will—even that favorite of hers which popped off two buttons when she tried to get into it.

But Mabel had one trump card. A month earlier for the first time George had taken her to a convention. The American Society of Personnel Officers was holding its annual clambake in New York. What a real adventure for her. They had even gone to a nightclub, where she realized she had no decent party dress. So while George was at the meetings she had, with much trepidation, walked over to Saks Fifth Avenue.

Adventures in Human Understanding

The elegant blue party gown she bought fit perfectly and looked magnificent on her—or so the sales clerk said. It had cost an outrageous price, which she had justified with undebatable feminine logic. She fully deserved it by virtue of all the savings she had made recently in the grocery bill. Mabel had concealed this from George, because the actual checks made out to the grocer were just as large as usual. But she had hidden the change she got back in a secret place—under the sink. That dress she had kept concealed in the back closet for just such an occasion as this "crab-date" at the Elk's.

When George left for work that morning she also didn't mention she planned a trip to the hairdresser in the afternoon. But when he got home that evening, Mabel was ready for him. All of a sudden he saw an attractive vision in blue, smiling at him with her hair neatly coiffured. It was like being transported back to the Senior Prom. Astonished, he gasped, "Wow! Is this my wife?" The hug and kiss that followed were longer than any in many years.

From then on through the rest of the evening everything coasted uphill. The meal, wonderful. The swing band, divine. They even hadn't forgotten how to jitterbug. George left an unusually large tip. A year ago Mabel would have bawled him out for such a waste of money. She thought of it now, but paused, smiled and simply squeezed his hand.

Spring came late that year. It was seven months since Elizabeth's death. The only reminder was a large photo of her sitting on the table beside the wedding picture. A month before she was killed George had insisted they get the best photographer in town.

For some time now that matter of sleeping had been a problem. The one-foot distance between them, which had been required for Elizabeth, always reminded them of her absence, and sadness would return. This particular night George decided it was no longer necessary. Moving over into the middle of the bed he snuggled against Mabel.

Maybe it was because this was the closest they had been in years, or perhaps because of "the crab date" and dancing, or because they were just tired of being apart. Anyway, something happened, something that hadn't occurred for a long time. It wasn't a Mount St. Helens, or even like Old Faithful, which had erupted frequently during their honeymoon in Yellowstone Park. It didn't last long, and right afterward Mabel dozed off. But George lay there on his side, one arm over the shoulder of the sleeping Mabel with his entire body bathed in a rosy glow. He thought of many things.

George slept-in that morning. When he awoke he heard Mabel humming an old familiar ditty while she was mixing up a batch of waffle dough—his favorite breakfast. Although she made waffles infrequently there was generally one for him and two for her. This time he noticed she had put two on his plate and one on hers.

The words of a song drifted back to him, "Just Molly and me, and Baby makes Three. We're happy in My Blue Heaven." He paraphrased it a bit in his mind, "Just Mabel and Me—" but when he came to "Baby" he thought of "Lizzy." The great sadness was almost gone—almost, but not quite. George extracted a crumpled handkerchief from his pants pocket and wiped his nose.

Mabel looked up as he entered the kitchen. "George, you know those machines, where you walk like you are skiing. I saw one in a catalog the other day. I'd like to get it. The Doctor said I needed to exercise." A request like this was unheard-of by George. For a moment an old remark of his came to mind, "Her exercise? That'll be the day." Then another thought pushed it out. "Sure, we'll get it tomorrow." When it was delivered the next day it was put on the back porch—in the corner where Elizabeth's bed had been located.

A week later George ran into Wayne. "We haven't talked for quite a while. How about me taking you and Mabel to breakfast Sunday? Meet you at Ruby's place. Afterwards, come over to the house, and we'll turn on the TV and see if the 49ers can beat the Broncos."

The meal went well, but just before he picked up the bill Wayne blurted out, "What gives with you two? You act like a couple of teenagers, always hugging, smooching and holding hands. You sure weren't that way a year ago. Have you been seeing a therapist?"

"Of course not," snapped George. "Me see a shrink? No way!"

Not being too interested in men-talk, Mabel had missed the interchange. She had been observing a young mother at the next table trying desperately to shovel a spoonful of cereal into the mouth of an uncooperative baby who was spitting it out as fast as she shoved it in. She wanted to tell the young woman, "Don't try to force the child." Too many parents these days had no patience.

"What did you say, Wayne? I missed your remark."

"I said how come you two are so lovey-dovey these days, always hugging and holding hands? You didn't used to be this way. Did you spend some time with a therapist?"

Mabel's first reaction would have been like George's. Then she thought again. Smiling reflectively while slowly stirring her coffee, she replied, "Yes—maybe we did—maybe we did."

Ode to a Pussycat

John G. Watkins

Ah, Swirly Tail, what truths thou couldst relate.
Perhaps of fishy viands smooth, delectable to feline taste.
Or yowling at the moon in thy more lusty youth.
And nursing then the little balls of fur
Who must require protection from an oft uncaring world.

And when the roar of wintry squall sheathes all thy fief
With gleaming white, and plagues thy crouch with painful paws
Wilt halt the heart's desire to claim dominion once again
From birds and squirrels and e'en the neighbour's tabby cat?
Better wait 'til smiles anew the shining orb of spring
So haste thee back now in-a-doors to cuddle thy master's lap.
With purring dreams of happy times that caring does renew.

Ah! humans sad, who strive for greed and power,
They never know, like those who understand,
With wisdom from their cat
That happiness comes not from goods, great wealth or might.
But holding close to those we love, For each of us
Divine endowed, a universal right.

Thoughts of a Therapist: Analysis and Comment

Some marriages improve over time. The partners become closer. Others, beginning with equal romance and high hopes, deteriorate over the years. They have become prisoners. Because of habit, children, social pressures, economic necessity or fear of living alone they cannot escape. They exist in mutual misery.

Sometimes this unhappy development begins when the partners start taking each other for granted. The resulting frustrations increase as each blames the other. Accusations evolve into constant arguments. Daily confrontations over even the most trivial differences result in hateful battles. Name-calling erodes the sense of self-worth in each. A once-promising relationship dissolves in shambles of mutual unhappiness. Of such is the marriage of George and Mabel. Can anything be done about it?

The participants seem powerless to reverse the flow of contention unless some outside source intervenes. It could be formal counseling or therapy, where individual insight is encouraged and maladaptive behavior patterns changed. But George considers consulting "a shrink" insulting. He is not "crazy." In the case of George and Mabel this "outside" source must be something unexpected.

In addition to their quarrels with each other, George and Mabel have many outside frustrations: For George, lack of promotion at work and competition with a talented brother-in-law. For Mabel, the overwhelming housework of cleaning an unrealistically large house. Defeated, she simply lets it slide into deterioration inside and out. Although George is not the philandering type, she must contend with an attractive secretary at George's office. She worries. Like many unhappy people, Mabel also "over-eats" herself into obesity.

George receives support from an old high-school buddy, Wayne, and Mabel from her sister, Emily, who has an even more difficult husband with whom to contend.

Midst a storm a half-dead kitten is deposited on their porch. At first not welcomed, they are intrigued and keep her as a pet. In their need for love and relationship they both compete for the cat's affection—which it provides. The kitten serves as a "transitional object" which moves them closer to each other. Hostility tends to melt if we have a mutual friend.

Disaster strikes when the cat is killed in an accident. In the face of disasters, tornadoes, hurricanes, wars, etc. people are drawn together. George and Mabel mutually grieve their loss.

This togetherness seeps over other areas of their interaction as they share, firstly, memories of their pet, and then memories of their childhood rejections. This stage of their interaction is a kind of "couples therapy." They realize they have much in common.

George resumes "courting behavior," and Mabel responds. This culminates in "dates" and romancing in ways of foregone years. Finally they resume sleeping together and mutually shared sex.

George's buddy, "Wayne," notices the great change in their relationship. He is amazed how affectionate toward each other they have become. He wants to know "why" and confronts them. It must be because they have been seeing a therapist.

George denies this as ridiculous, but Mabel, more thoughtful, realizes that they have—but it is a furry little kitten who has changed their malevolent cycle into a constructive one.

Unhappy couples sometimes have a baby in the hope that this will bring them together. However, if this child is primarily sought as a solution to a bad marriage it may only make matters worse. It is the unexpected intervention that has the best opportunity for success.

Chapter 9

The Cuckoo Bird's Egg[1]

"Look at that mess on my carpet," shouted Roger, red-faced and enraged. He pointed to the large spot in the middle of the pale brown carpet while slapping Quentin repeatedly. "I told you to take Trixie out for a walk every morning after breakfast. I suppose you forgot to, you lazy brat."

The cowering 7-year-old was crying, "But Daddy, I did take her out. I did take her out. She just had to do it again."

Roger increased the vehemence of his slapping. "And I've told you a thousand times that when you lie to me you're really going to get it."

"But Daddy, I'm not lying. I did take her out. I did take her out," begged Quentin. Grabbing his hair and shielding his face with his arms he tried desperately to escape the barrage of blows. Finally, bursting free, he rushed screaming from the room, hoping to hide in the upstairs closet.

Melanie, who couldn't stand it when Roger was in one of his violent spells, had already scurried out the back door and, holding both hands over her ears, sat helplessly on the bottom step. She always felt sorry for Quentin in times like these, but she also felt incapable of doing anything about it. Nobody ever stood up to Roger when he was angry. Sometimes, but not often, she would comfort Quentin providing Roger didn't see her "coddling that boy."

Roger had just returned home after an unhappy day at the Chevrolet agency where he was a sales representative. One old

---

[1] The cuckoo bird lays its egg in the nest of other birds who then must assume responsibility for its hatching and feeding.

Adventures in Human Understanding

used car, no new car sales. When he discovered the wet spot on the carpet of his study he instantly swung into action, grabbing Quentin and laying it on before asking any questions.

When something went wrong in the Higgins household Roger knew instinctively that Quentin was to blame. He had felt that way since the blonde-haired baby had been born. Everybody else in the family, he, Melanie and their first born, James, were dark haired.

Roger never could quite overcome a feeling of inferiority toward his younger brother, Edward, who was a good two inches taller. Furthermore, following graduation from Dartmouth, Edward had been given a position as "Administrative Assistant" in their father's firm. Roger was convinced it was because of favoritism toward Edward.

As a child Roger had never liked blonde kids—ever since Ole Nelson beat up on him in the fourth grade. Aage Peterson and other sixth grade kids had sneered and taunted him. He swore then he would get "that damned Swede" some day.

In high school the more attractive girls had tended to gravitate toward Edward. So when Melanie, a gentle, dark-haired beauty, had shown an interest in him he maintained his best behavior and persuaded her to accept his proposal of marriage.

Some in the family wondered whether he would be a good family man. However, the day his eldest son, James, was born Roger was very pleased and proud. He decided the boy would be named "James" after his own father—providing the second name was "Roger," to which Melanie agreed. So James Roger Higgins entered the household, the apple of his father's eye.

During the following nine years Roger and his son, James, had been pals. Baseball, fishing, hunting rabbits. Roger put up a ring on the front of the garage, and they would play basketball in the evenings after Roger returned from work. "Jim" would run to meet his Dad at five o'clock each afternoon and often be carried home on Roger's shoulder. Melanie appreciated their camaraderie.

The Cuckoo Bird's Egg

But when Quentin arrived, two years after Jim, Roger's mood seemed to change. He was irritable and would seldom smile. Occasional outbursts of rage burst forth, especially when he disciplined Quentin—in ways that Melanie felt were unnecessarily severe. Roger stayed many hours at the office, while Melanie was sick much of the time. Quentin was left to play by himself.

One day a long white van came to the house, and two men in white coats carried the boy's mother out of the house on a stretcher. His father explained to Quentin that his mother had cancer, and that she might not come back, then added: "Maybe if you'd been a better boy she wouldn't have gotten sick." Quentin was crushed.

A month later the entire family: Quentin; Roger; Jim; Roger's younger brother, Edward; Edward's wife, Anne; and Roger's father, Grandpa James; were together as they buried Melanie.

Quentin felt that somehow he was responsible for his mother's death and stayed out of Roger's way whenever possible. However, he couldn't seem to escape the constant criticisms and angry accusations of his father. Melanie had been a gentle person and was endeared by the other family members. Tears flowed in profusion at the funeral. Quentin wondered why his father didn't cry.

A week later the family suffered another blow. Quentin's grandfather, James Sr., while on a trip inspecting his properties, was killed in a car accident. Although Quentin had admired Grandpa James, they were not close. To Quentin this tall athletically built giant with the dark, slightly grayed hair was a figure of awe. He sensed that Grandpa was very important to all the family.

James Higgins, Senior, was an investment broker and reputed to be quite wealthy. He had a suite of offices in a tall building downtown. Edward had an office next to his father's.

At 28 years of age, Edward, a tall, well-built man with light brown hair, had married Anne immediately after getting the job. She was a slender, neatly dressed young woman, with wavy-smooth blonde hair. Their friends agreed that Edward and Anne had a good marriage.

A few days after Grandpa's death the family met in the living room of Roger's house to hear a reading of the will.

Michael Thompson, Esq., senior partner in the firm of Thompson and Billings, weighed nearly 300 pounds. It was distributed more East and West than North and South and completely filled the large relaxing chair plus spilling over the arm-rests. His ample handlebar moustache wiggled up and down while he pontificated the many small bequests first. These were followed by substantial bequests to both Roger and Edward.

Roger, who had been dozing through much of these, roused to attention-alert when he heard Lawyer Thompson read: "I wish my younger son, Edward, who has been associated with my business affairs, to act as Administrator of my estate and to hold Power of Attorney for disbursing these bequests in the interest of my heirs. No bond is to be required as I have complete trust in him."

Roger was greatly irked and on the edge of getting angry. "Why was I not appointed Administrator of the estate? I'm his oldest son." Mr. Thompson re-read that item, then looking Roger straight in the eye, he stated in a slow and firm voice: "Your father was in sound health, physically and mentally, when he dictated the terms of his will to me four months ago. He knew exactly how he wanted to dispose of his assets and whom he wanted as Administrator of his estate."

Roger slunk back in his chair and was silent. The reading of the long and complex will continued.

Finally the attorney came to a passage which surprised no one. "And to my two grandchildren, Quentin and James Roger Higgins, I leave the remainder of my estate, which is to be divided equally between them."

Mr. Thompson coughed loudly, cleared his throat and wiped his forehead with a wrinkled handkerchief before continuing. It was a hot day in the middle of an Indian summer, and his excess poundage was protesting.

Edward and his wife Anne knew why this part of the will did not pertain to them. They had hoped for children. Anne had been reared in a family with three brothers and four sisters, She confidently expected to have a similar one. During their courtship Edward had confided in her that he intended to name their first son "James Higgins" after the father whom he so admired. He knew his Dad would like that.

However, after Roger and Melanie had named their first son "James," Edward gave up on that dream. There would be too many "James Higgins"s in the family.

His frustration grew during the following nine years as Anne never conceived. She felt that somehow she had disappointed Edward. They had gone to a fertility clinic and followed all the directions, but with no result. Now they were almost reconciled to being childless, and there was no more talk about it. The mention of grandchildren in his father's will, however, rekindled a feeling of sadness in Edward's mind.

Mr. Thompson continued reading the will. "There is an addendum he dictated to me a month ago that he insisted be included. It is as follows:

'I, James Higgins, want to be assured that these funds will be inherited by only those grandchildren who are my biological heirs. If either of them should prove not to be, then the inheritance will accrue completely to the other.'"

A hush enveloped the room. Everyone looked at Quentin, then at Roger and then back at Quentin again.

It was Roger who first broke the silence.

"I knew it. I've always suspected it, and Dad knew it too. Melanie and I were estranged the year before Quentin was born, and I've never felt he was my son. I'm sure she was playing around. Once I mentioned my suspicion to Father, but at that time he wouldn't consider it seriously. Quentin doesn't take after the Higgins family. I guess it finally had to come out. So Jim gets the entire remainder, yes?"

Quentin, even though only seven, understood. Fighting back tears he rushed from the room. He didn't want to live anymore, not with a father who hated him, nor with the rest of them who didn't even care. Edward's wife. Anne, recognizing the child's despair, got up quickly and left. A few minutes later she found him sobbing in his little "safe room," the upstairs closet, where he had crawled into a corner.

"I'm here, Honey. There are people who love you and will not let you stay alone."

Anne cradled the weeping child, who within a week had lost his mother and now was abandoned by his father. He was alone in a world that didn't want him.

Between sobs Quentin lifted his voice. "Will Daddy throw me out of the house, now that he says he's not my father?"

Anne's gentle voice soothed as he clung to her. "You stay with us until we find what's going to happen. We love you."

She had no idea what would happen now. Would Quentin become a ward of the court, adopted out to some strange family? Would he ever surmount the terrible rejection by his father? She only knew he was a lonely little orphan boy, and she, who had never been able to have a child, needed to mother him.

Back in the living room, the other members of the family were recovering from the shock of Quentin's sudden departure. Clearing his throat, downing a glass of water, and obviously trying to regain his composure, Mr. Thompson began explaining further the terms of the will.

"That remainder, which is to be divided between the biological grandchildren of James Higgins, Senior, comes to—uh—let me see," Mr. Thompson lowered his glasses and peered at an important-looking document. "It's about 500,000 dollars."

Roger smiled. His son would appreciate the good, fatherly care he had given over the years. He knew Jim would be generous with his inheritance, and he was already thinking of a bigger place necessary to house both himself and Jim.

"Can you simply make out the check to James today?"

"Well no," replied the corpulent attorney. "A judge has to make the decision. I'll schedule it for probate court."

The family members filed out in a daze. Jim was pleased with the bequests, but he felt a sadness and an emptiness. Over the years he had sensed his father's rejection of Quentin. Even though he had been the recipient of Roger's favoritism, he felt sorry for Quentin, and only wished that his Dad would be kinder to his little brother.

Hoping to make up for his father's mistreatment of Quentin, Jim had come to the rescue of his sibling many times—like when an older boy had seized Quentin's new bicycle and wouldn't give it back. Jim had responded promptly to Quentin's cries. He came running, had confronted the bully, and forced him to return the bike. It made Quentin feel good that somebody cared about him.

"Thanks, Jim. Butch is too big. He was going to hit me."

Jim had never experienced his father's wrath personally. Realizing the implications of the will, the 9-year-old wanted to be with his young brother, but he was afraid that his father would get angry if he was seen near Quentin.

Two weeks later the family assembled in the county courthouse. Judge McDonald had asked that all members be present when the will was probated, primarily because of that matter regarding the grandchildren.

Roger appeared first, leading Jim by the hand. They took seats in the front. He was in an expansive mood, nodding, smiling and chatting with all around him.

Adventures in Human Understanding

Edward and Anne, with Quentin at their side, arrived soon afterward and sat down several rows back. Roger ignored them. About a dozen other individuals were present, bored and impatiently waiting for some personally relevant case.

Quentin sensed that something significant was about to happen. He was very impressed when the black-robed judge appeared. His Honor, the Judge, still had a few wisps of red hair remaining on the almost-bald brow. His features were stern, but an occasional twinkle in his eyes suggested he could still appreciate a lighter moment.

In a loud and stentorious voice, the bailiff, a short, brown-suited pipsqueak, announced, "Everybody stand." Clearing his throat, he then proclaimed, "The first case on the docket is the probate of the will of Mr. James Higgins, Senior, deceased."

With difficulty, Mr. Thompson pushed his chair back from the table, struggled to his feet, and ambled his 295 pounds toward the judge.

"Your Honor. Last week when I presented the Higgins Will for probate, you noted the provision made by Mr. James Higgins, Senior, regarding the paternity of his two grandchildren. And you requested that I have DNA tests applied to Mr. Roger Higgins and his two sons, Quentin and James. I have had these tests run, and I would like to call to the stand Mr. Gregory Oglethorpe, Director of Western Labs, Inc."

Roger nodded at the judge and smiled.

A rather spindly, thin individual, who might have been a character from a Dickens novel, shuffled to the witness stand and plunked himself down on the straight-backed wooden chair.

"Do you promise to tell the truth, the whole truth and only the truth, so help you God?" proclaimed the bailiff, holding forth a Bible. The witness thrust out a skinny and trembling hand, then replied almost in a whisper. "I do."

Mr. Oglethorpe's voice was so weak and indistinct that both Roger and Edward had to lean forward to hear. The attorney asked the question a second time and then admonished Mr. Oglethorpe to speak louder.

"State your name and occupation," he queried.

The witness raised his voice almost to pianissimo. He gazed blankly at the judge for several seconds. "Gregory P. Oglethorpe. I am Director of the Western Labs. We perform medical tests for purposes of diagnosis in legal cases."

Roger frowned. He was not impressed with Mr. Oglethorpe. There was something about this witness that gave him a feeling of uneasiness.

"Does that include DNA testing?"

"It does."

"Are you accredited to do such testing?"

"We are certified by the American Association of Blood Banks."

"How many years have you been administering these tests?"

Mr. Oglethorpe thumbed through some notes he had brought. "Six—no, seven."

"Are there any questions regarding the competence of this expert witness?"

The room was silent. Roger, somewhat reassured, leaned back in his chair. Edward stared straight ahead at the witness while Mr. Oglethorpe explained in a monotonous whisper the pros and cons of DNA analysis, including the validating research.

Even the judge had to ask him several times to repeat his answer to Mr. Thompson's questions.

Adventures in Human Understanding

"You were requested to secure DNA samples from Mr. Roger Higgins and from his two sons, Quentin and Jim. Is that correct?"

Anne moved over on the bench and put her arms around Quentin. Sensing that something important was about to happen, and being frightened, Quentin huddled close to her, reassured by the warmth of her body.

"And can you say that it is possible to determine paternity with a high degree of accuracy in a case like this?"

"When we have obtained adequate samples, and the results are definite, like within a 1 to 1000 chance of error, we can state with overwhelming probability that a given donor is or is not the parent of a given child."

"And have you secured such verification in the case of Roger Higgins and his two sons?"

"We have."

Roger turned around and smiled at Edward and Anne. It was the broadest smile she had seen on him in years.

"We find that Quentin Higgins is definitely, beyond any reasonable doubt, the biological son of Roger Higgins."

A look of unbelieving consternation crept over the countenance of Roger—like the shadow of a solar eclipse sweeping the landscape. The enormity of his possible mistake regarding Quentin began to surge through him. But even as he started to experience self-doubts, his anger reacted. How dare this shrimp of a lab technician contradict his years of observation and knowledge. He must be incompetent. With great difficulty Roger controlled his mounting rage while waiting for the next bit of testimony.

"And have you examined the DNA samples of James Roger Higgins as compared to those of the father, Roger Higgins?"

The Cuckoo Bird's Egg

"We have, and we find that the child named James, and called 'Jim,' is probably not the son of Roger Higgins. The DNA findings are quite clear."

A roar exploded from the front row.

"You lying son-of-a-bitch. Where did you learn to be a DNA examiner? In grade school? Your Honor, must we put up with such incompetence?"

Judge McDonald pounded his gavel. "Order in the courtroom. If that man speaks further, remove him."

Roger stood up and, after a dagger-filled look at the witness, he strode from the room. Edward followed Roger, hoping to quiet his brother before rage got him in real trouble, maybe even being jailed for contempt of court.

Both of the boys were now crying. Jim ran back to Anne and hugged close to her and Quentin.

There being no opposing attorney to cross-examine him, the witness was dismissed.

The Judge was about to issue a final decree stating that Quentin was the only biological son of Roger and that accordingly all of the "remaining" funds would be issued in trust to him, with his uncle, Edward Higgins, granted power of attorney. At that point Mr. Thompson approached the judge and said, "Your Honor, the members of the Higgins family are obviously disturbed over the testimony of this witness. May I request a recess while I confer with them?"

"Granted. The court will recess for 30 minutes."

Half an hour later the attorney again addressed the court.

"Your Honor, Mr. Roger Higgins believes the DNA tests were incompetently administered. He intends to initiate suit against the Western Labs. In view of this problem within the family I request that decision on probating the will of Mr. James Higgins, Senior, be

Adventures in Human Understanding

deferred until further DNA testing by another laboratory can be secured."

The Judge thought for a moment and then announced: "Final probate of this will will be deferred until October 27th, two weeks from today. Additional DNA tests will be administered by a laboratory which is acceptable both to Mr. Roger Higgins and to you as counsel for the estate of Mr. James Higgins, Senior."

The judge pounded his gavel. "Court is hereby adjourned for today."

Anne took the two boys home, while Roger and Edward repaired to Mr. Thompson's office to consider the next step.

Edward had cornered Roger in the hall and managed to get him calmed down. However, he was most vehement in his denunciation of Mr. Oglethorpe. "That lying son-of-a bitch, what's he trying to get away with? We'll sue him for a million dollars for malpractice, falsifying test results—Yeah, and another million for inflicting damage and shame on my son, James. Can we do it?"

"Yes, you can," replied Mr. Thompson, "but since I represent the estate, you will have to secure another lawyer to represent you in this suit."

"Give us a recommendation. Come on, Edward, let's get that other lawyer and sue the bastard for everything he's got."

Edward looked rather hesitant.

"Roger. This is between you and that lab director. Anne and I are taking no position."

"No position. Hell. Can't you support your own brother? Did I ever let you down?"

Edward tried to be calm and disagree without antagonizing Roger into one of his violent spells.

"Suppose the lab tests were not incompetent. Suppose the new tests come out the same way. Then what?"

A look of astonishment appeared on Roger's face.

"You don't take those findings seriously, do you?"

"Maybe not, but I would prefer to wait and see. There will be plenty of time to initiate a suit afterward. We'll cooperate with you in securing a completely competent and fair lab."

"Well, I'm going to sue the bastard, even if you won't support your own brother."

Roger exited rapidly, slamming the door. Edward and the attorney were left staring at one another. Meanwhile Anne had taken the two boys to her house.

The Edward Higgins domicile was conservatively attractive. A two-story colonial, painted pale blue and trimmed in white, it was located near the end of a private road sided by similar homes. Collectively these homes demonstrated in no uncertain terms that well-to-do people, successful in business or the professions, occupied this suburb. A luxury van or station wagon was parked on many driveways fronting the two-car garages. Between the one-half acre lots and behind the homes one could see that most, with the exception of the Higgins's place, sported playground equipment.

Quentin and Jim had often enjoyed a visit to "Uncle Edward's place," and immediately bounced up the white-painted stairs to the spare room in which they had occasionally slept—sent there by Melanie when Roger was in one of his foul moods. Anne allowed them much freedom but did not tolerate dirty shoes and insisted that they clean up the room before they returned home to Roger's more modest abode.

October 27th was rather frosty but clear. Morning had seemed to dawn earlier than usual. Edward and Anne had been awake since 6:30 getting the two boys bathed and cleaned up for another court appearance. Anne did not want them to appear before the judge unless hands were washed, hair was combed and they were wearing unwrinkled white shirts. Obviously unaware of the drama that might be unfolding, or of its significance for their future lives, they had been giggling and teasing one another. It required some effort to get them both corralled.

At fifteen minutes to ten Roger and the other Higgins family members appeared in the courtroom. Roger ignored Edward, but smiled at Anne and, judging that her presence would be reassuring, permitted Jim to sit with her and Quentin.

Anne had always been recognized by the family as the opposite in temperament from Roger. Whenever she was present an aura of peacefulness descended. Everybody felt secure. People did not criticize one another, and there was little disagreement. To the contrary, whenever Roger entered a room, the air would be filled with contention. Squabbling and disparaging remarks burgeoned.

But today Roger was calm and friendly. He knew that his position would be proven to all, and he looked forward to suing "that bastard" into bankruptcy. Once more he was smiling.

The court was called to order as usual. Everybody stood, including the two little boys whose playful interactions were somewhat subdued by the solemnity of the occasion. They would probably remember this day for many years in the future.

The judge began the session by asking Mr. Thompson a question:

"The probate of the will of Mr. James Higgins, Senior, was to be concluded today following the report by an independent laboratory concerning further DNA tests on Mr. Roger Higgins and his sons, Quentin and James. Was a laboratory selected that met the approval of both yourself and Mr. Roger Higgins?"

"Yes, Your Honor. After considering several accredited firms within the city offering DNA testing, Mr. Roger Higgins and I agreed on the Tri-State Laboratories, which is fully accredited. Before agreement was reached, and at the insistence of Mr. Roger Higgins, I personally accompanied him and his brother, Mr. Edward Higgins, to interview its Director." Roger nodded. They

The Cuckoo Bird's Egg

had visited two other labs, which were rejected by Roger for reasons he couldn't quite specify, but he seemed impressed with the third, headed by a Mr. Palmer.

Ronald J. Palmer was 6 foot 3 inches in height—almost as tall as Roger's father had been. About 45 years of age and with clean-cut features, he spoke in a very confident-sounding voice. Roger had tried to get Mr. Palmer to admit that DNA testing was very controversial and not well-validated by scientific researchers. In contrast to the others they interviewed, this lab director had patiently listened to all of Roger's reservations and did not argue with him. Although he had not always agreed with Roger, he had answered each question simply and clearly. Roger was impressed. With a sense of closure, he had finally declared, "That's the one we want." Both Edward and Mr. Thompson agreed. Accordingly, Tri-State Laboratories was selected to run the final validating tests.

In court, the initial questioning went much as before. Mr. Palmer had answered all the questions put to him by the lawyer, including a few clarifying ones asked by the judge, such as whether he was aware that there had been a previous set of tests and had been told their findings.

"Your Honor. I knew that previous DNA tests had been made. I did not know what lab had administered them. I understood they were controversial, but I was not told their conclusions. We obtained good-sized DNA samples, and I must say that Mr. Higgins and the two boys cooperated fully."

Roger smiled. Throughout the courtroom there was an air of expectant tension. Because of the drama at the end of the prior meeting, the case had attracted local attention, and two news reporters were present eagerly hoping for excitement. They would probably be disappointed. The judge, through Mr. Thompson, had extracted a promise from Roger to control his temper on pain of being punished for contempt of court.

The usual preliminaries were concluded. And now the crucial questions were asked—this time by the judge.

Adventures in Human Understanding

"Mr. Palmer, have you reached a conclusion regarding the paternity of Quentin Higgins and James Roger Higgins?"

"We have, your honor. In the case of Quentin Higgins we find that Mr. Roger Higgins is almost certainly his father. In the case of James Higgins, Jr. we find that Mr. Roger Higgins is probably not his father."

The explosion that burst from the first row this time could be compared only to the impact of a tornado. Roger, his face a fiery red, and with tears streaming down his cheeks, thrashed the air with his fist. Shouting vulgarities, he headed for the exit. Quentin and Jim, who were completely bored with the questioning, had been pushing one another out into the aisle. Startled by the furor, they were now desperately scrambling to reach the safety of Anne's waiting arms. Roger shoved them roughly aside: "Get the hell out of my way, you little bastards."

"Arrest that man," shouted Judge McDonald toward the Sergeant at Arms who was pursuing Roger out the door of the courtroom. Trailing behind were the two reporters, one with a camera.

"Order in the courtroom! Order in the courtroom!" demanded the judge, pounding his gavel.

Gradually the hubbub and general confusion quieted down. Edward appeared to be paralyzed and in a state of shock. However, Anne stood up. "You stay with your Uncle Edward," she exclaimed to the two boys. "Your Honor, may I speak to you?"

Judge McDonald had recovered from this moment of disruption. He was not accustomed to having a person in the audience approach him. However, he recognized Anne as a member of the family, and had been impressed by the quiet and efficient manner in which she had replied to several questions directed toward her once when in another case of his she had served as a witness.

"Your Honor. The probate of this will has been an extremely emotional trauma to all members of our family. May I make a few observations which would help all of us cope with this crisis?" She didn't use the word "suggestions" to a judge, but that was what she was hoping to present.

Judge McDonald had always been a stickler for decorum and the proper conduct of legal protocol in his court. But for once the warm human being emerged that lay behind his strict judicial demeanor.

"Proceed."

"Your Honor. My brother-in-law Mr. Roger Higgins is a sick man. We who know him and love him have recognized his emotional deterioration for the past nine years. He alternates between calmness and spells of uncontrollable rage. My husband, his brother, and I have been planning to get him professional psychiatric help, but we've been waiting until the proper time. I know that he has offended the decorum of the court, but we ask your understanding and leniency."

"His Honor" looked a bit amused. He realized that she wanted to give him "suggestions" as to how he should judge the case. It was quite irregular, but he was not offended.

"In addition, Sir, in view of my brother-in-law's temporary emotional incapacity, my husband, Edward, and I request that you grant custody of the two boys to us, both Quentin and James Higgins. We have a large house, a spare bedroom and are financially prepared to assume this responsibility."

All this was not according to normal court procedure, but Judge McDonald, who had presided at innumerable bitter family fights, could recognize a promising solution when he saw one. With little hesitation he decided: "Sentence will be not be pronounced on Roger Higgins at this time for his unseemly outbursts in court, but I want a report within the next month as to what psychiatric evaluation or treatment has been administered to him."

"This won't be easy," thought Edward, realizing what Roger's reaction would be at a suggestion that he get a psychiatric evaluation. "Oh well, we'll have to worry about that later."

The judge continued. "Temporary custody of the two boys, Quentin Higgins and James Roger Higgins, is awarded to Mr. Edward Higgins and his wife, Anne."

Then after a few questions to Mr. Thompson, the judge issued another decision.

"In the pending probate case Mr. Edward Higgins will serve as Administrator for the estate of James Higgins, Senior, and is authorized to make disbursements to the designated heirs as provided in the will. Mr. Edward Higgins is also granted Power of Attorney over the funds in Trust bequeathed by James Higgins, Senior, to his grandson, Quentin Higgins, and is authorized to withdraw from the Trust such funds as are necessary to provide for the health and welfare of said Quentin Higgins. Court is adjourned."

Even Judge McDonald was sweating. With a sigh of relief he retreated to his inner chambers. It had been quite a day.

There was a chill in the air that evening. Edward, feeling the need for peace and quiet, had built a fire in the small fireplace within his study. An atmosphere of "following-the-storm" pervaded the room. Everybody seemed to feel a need for togetherness. Anne reclined in the easy chair which, like the couch, she had tastefully chosen in a matching brown leather. The two boys were laughing and rolling on that couch. Edward was watching them while sitting quietly on the swivel chair in front of his large oak desk. He chuckled. The boys resembled the two bear cubs that had so amused him and Anne during last year's vacation in Glacier Park.

Edward, musing over the day's events, kept returning to Anne's talk with the judge. He felt an overwhelming wave of emotion as he looked at her simple but pleasant features. At that moment she seemed to him the most wonderful woman in the world. He was overwhelmed with both respect and love.

It was difficult to keep tears from coming down as he recalled that day, years ago, he had proposed to her. It was a frosty night, much like this evening. He was walking her back to the dorm at the College. The question suddenly popped out. They had been dating for some time, so her answer did not really surprise him. But by making a mutual commitment, something new had been added. In a month he had graduated and they were married. Now he experienced the same feelings, but today they were much richer, much deeper. He wanted to take her in his arms and tell her about all this again, but the yearnings were so overwhelming he couldn't speak.

The only thing that came to his mind was a recollection of an old TV program he had watched as a child. It was a funny program, but at the end of each episode a fat man had embraced his long-suffering wife and announced, "Baby, you're the greatest." Over and over he thought, "You're the greatest. You're the greatest."

Anne looked up from her reading and announced. "I'm very tired. Think I'll get ready for bed." When she came over and kissed him "good night," he could say nothing but only cling to her a little longer than usual before she pulled away. She disappeared upstairs, carrying the book on "Gardens for the Home" with her.

After she had gone Edward looked at his watch.

"Time for bed, you rascals."

The two boys stopped their wrestling. Jim, still quite alert and wanting to stall off bedtime, issued a dare.

"Bet I can hide, and you can't find me."

Quentin had been learning that you had to stand up to a challenge.

"I can find you. I can find you."

Jim bounded up the stairs. Edward expected Quentin to follow immediately, but Quentin had something important to say, something he needed to ask.

"Uncle Ed, did Grandpa give me a lot of money—all for me?"

Adventures in Human Understanding

"Yes, he did, Quentin."

"Well, can I use it to buy candy and anything I want?"

This called for diplomacy and some child psychology. "Probably, but the judge says that you and I have to agree it's O.K. for you to spend the money that way. How about it?"

Quentin was quickly appeased.

"Fine with me. But why did Daddy say that he wasn't my father? Isn't he my father?"

"Yes, Quentin, he really is. But your Daddy is sick, and he gets confused."

"If he is sick, does that mean he'll go away and not come back, like Mama?"

"No, I don't think he's going to stay away. He'll be back."

Quentin had one more question puzzling him. "Did Grandpa give money to Jim too?

"No. I'm sorry, he didn't."

"Well then, Uncle Ed, can I give some of my money to Jim? He's my good friend."

Now Edward really had trouble holding the tears back.

"The judge has to agree, but, yes, I think we can arrange it."

He was thinking about all of the laws regarding gifts, and how much he could authorize from Quentin's trust as Power of Attorney. "Now run along and see if you can find Jim." Quentin dashed up the stairs.

Edward sat quietly staring at the flames in the fireplace. Soon after he was startled by a joyous squeal from upstairs.

The Cuckoo Bird's Egg

"I see you. I know you're there. Come out. I win. I win."

This was followed by peals of laughter. Edward settled back in quiet contemplation. He sat there a long time. The flames in the fireplace got lower and lower. The noises and giggling that had been emanating from the boys' bedroom ceased. He felt alone and at peace.

Finally, stirring himself, he turned to the big oak desk. Pulling a small drawer open and reaching back into it he extracted a blue-colored envelope. He knew who the letter was from and what it might contain. It had arrived many days ago, but with all the confusion of his father's death, the probate of the will, and the court appearances, he had set it aside to await a time when he could calmly read and digest it. This was his first moment of privacy. With mixed feelings of eagerness and anxiety he opened it and read:

"Edward Dearest: In a few days I will be gone. I am not afraid to go. Perhaps I have completed what I was sent here for. Do you remember that night over ten years ago when you were in college? I knocked on the door of your student apartment. Roger was in a terrible rage—over what, I don't know, but he had hit me many times on the face. I realized then that he was not the man I thought I had married. I didn't know what to do or where to go, so I just blindly ran to your apartment. You were his brother, and you had always treated me with respect.

"I remember you wiped away my tears, calmed me down and held me. I felt then like I was a little girl, and I hugged you. I told you that Roger had stormed away and said he wouldn't be back until morning. Then, Dear, I kissed you, and you responded to me. I needed a closeness and a warmth I never experienced with Roger. I also knew then that I had married the wrong man, that I loved you, that I wanted you, that I needed you.

"Roger was strong and persistent. I was attracted to him. At the time he seemed glamorous, while you were more unassuming, quiet and steady. I didn't realize before that night how much I needed steadiness.

Adventures in Human Understanding

"Then, Dear, do you remember that we felt closer and closer as the night went on until we truly belonged to each other.

"When I left, just before daylight, I thought I should feel guilty. But I didn't. I had been loved by the man I loved, and Roger by his brutality had sacrificed any loyalty I owed him.

"Well Darling, as you may have guessed, we started a new little life. When Jim came I wondered how Roger would react. I even thought of divorcing him, hoping I could win you. But he was good to Jim right from the start, and later that year you became engaged to Anne. I decided to let well enough alone.

"I never could understand why Roger was such a good father to Jim and treated Quentin, his own child, so badly. Often I wanted to rescue Quentin, but I was never strong enough. Maybe that's why I was sick so much of the time. I never told you that Jim was our son, but I suspect you knew."

Edward put the letter down and mused to himself for a few moments, "Yes, I suspected, and guess I probably also knew, but I was never sure." He resumed reading the letter.

"And now, Dear, I am reconciled to leaving. It is not every woman who is privileged to have a baby with the man she loves. I hope Roger's anger will never turn toward Jim, but if it does, please take care of our son and see that he is protected. He will grow to be the kind of man you are. Just remember, Darling, that I love you and have always loved you.

"Melanie"

Edward sat a long time thinking. The flames in the fireplace no longer reached up toward the chimney. There were only a few embers remaining—glowing red embers. Edward stood up and strolling slowly over to the fireplace he gently placed the letter on those embers. Afterwards, he sat down on the floor and stared at the glow until it ceased entirely.

It was almost an hour later when he realized he should check the locks on the front and back doors. Then he walked upstairs and down the hall. As he passed the room where the boys were silently sleeping he thought, "Maybe Anne and I can have a family after all."

Thoughts of a Therapist: Analysis and Comment

Roger Higgins is a very angry and unstable man. He believes his wife, Melanie, has been unfaithful to him. He takes his rage out on his second son, Quentin (age 7), whom he thinks is the offspring of another man. Roger's wife, Melanie, feels helpless in the face of his anger at Quentin. She cannot protect the boy. Melanie is often sick, and develops a fatal cancer which has strong psychosomatic overtones.

"Possession" of one's spouse and jealousy of one's paternal right is a common issue among men. This stems from the tremendous motivation among males to prove masculinity and male potency. The drive is clearly manifested after puberty when competition in sports is high. Witness the strivings of Eldridge in the *Flagpole* story. Fathering a child is socially considered as proof of a man's masculinity, and the custody of children is a common issue in divorce suits. Roger has to cope with poor results in his sales job. He also feels inferior to his younger brother, Edward, who is more successful financially. In their rivalry, Roger's one superiority over his brother is his ability to produce a child. If he had known that Edward was the source of the humiliation, re: his presumed illegitimate son, violence might have broken out in the family. Edward and Anne have always wanted a family with children of their own, but this has been denied them. Infertile couples often exhaust medical possibilities and then compulsively seek to adopt a child through black-market contacts or through visits to Russia, Romania, etc. where there are many abandoned children.

When Roger's wife, Melanie, dies the family mourns at her funeral. Shortly afterward, the patriarchal father of Roger and Edward dies, leaving a substantial inheritance. A successful businessman, he designated Edward as the Administrator of his estate—much to the disgust of Roger.

Adventures in Human Understanding

The will specifies that a substantial portion of the inheritance will be divided equally between his two grandchildren, Quentin and James Roger Higgins, Jr. (age 9), called Jim. If either of the boys proves not to be the grandfather's biological grandchild, the entire amount will go to the other. Here again we see the importance males place on being the biological father of their children (and grandchildren).

Roger immediately seizes on this provision to proclaim his conviction that Quentin is not his child and to demand the money now go to his son, Jim. The lawyer explains that a court will make this decision. Quentin, devastated by his father's rejection, runs and hides in a closet. He is consoled by Anne.

In court, the judge rules that a DNA examination must be made of Quentin, Jim and Roger to determine paternity. The DNA specialist reports that Quentin is the biological child of Roger, but that Jim is not. Infuriated, Roger runs from the room vowing to sue the specialist for incompetence.

People who have committed themselves to a belief often adamantly refuse to accept its disproof. Witness the resistance to accepting the findings of science regarding evolution—and for a few even that the earth is round.

The judge rules that a second DNA examination will be made by another specialist agreeable to all. This second finding confirms the first. Whereupon Roger, completely unable to accept these results, rejects both children, and rushes away in a state of violent rage. If the findings were true, then he would have to face his seven-year mistreatment of his own son. Anne, the diplomat in the family, prevails on the judge to accept that Roger is mentally ill and needs psychiatric treatment. The judge then awards temporary custody of both children to Anne and Edward.

After Anne and the children have gone to bed, Edward, in the privacy of his study, reads a hidden letter from Melanie written just before she died. In it, she reveals that Edward is the real father of Jim. She asks him to take care of "our son." The letter also shows that Jim, as well as Quentin, is a biological grandchild of James Roger Higgins, Sr., conceived by Edward before he married Anne.

(Coincidentally Jim has been named, according to Edward's dream, after the grandfather.)

However, for family harmony Edward will keep this secret and arrange from his position of Estate Administrator to use the legacy for the benefit of both boys—an ethical position the legality of which could be questioned. Some day it may be desirable to reveal to Jim that he, Edward, not Roger, is Jim's real father, but it might create a difficult problem for Jim, since Jim had enjoyed a good father-son relationship with Roger.

The close emotional bonding between the two lads (in spite of their differential treatment by Roger) is touchingly revealed. Unlike the competitiveness of Roger and Edward, Quentin and Jim will be supportive brothers to each other.

With a sense of closure, Edward realises that now he and Anne can have a family of their own. In the happy ending, a family of loving, well-adjusted parents is established. They will provide a stable home for the two boys, and meet both Anne's and Edward's need for children.

Although people often marry for sex and companionship needs, society established the institution of marriage, with its legal and religious sanction, primarily to protect children during their long period of dependency.

Furthermore, women generally seek mates (consciously or unconsciously) who will provide favorable genetic inheritance and protection for them and their children. Witness the case of Madonna in the story of The Novel. In today's marriage marketplace, economic power often is valued more than physical strength.

The story achieves a socially desirable solution to a difficult and secretive family problem. It leaves unresolved whether the unstable, maladjusted brother, Roger, receives effective therapy and overcomes his emotional problems.

Part III

The Autumn of Life

Chapter 10

Andrew and his Old Sheepdog

I was sitting on one end of the park bench looking across the deep blue lake at the impressive hulk of Mt. Rainier in the distance. Dark green, it presided over the landscape. Its huddled little patches of snow guarding the valleys in this early fall were waiting for their winter reinforcements. So calm and peaceful, not a single wisp of wind. Even the small blotches of white that slowly paddled by in the lake gave nary a quack.

The ivory-colored buildings in this forested lake-front park had been built by Uncle Sam to provide a home for those soldiers and sailors who could no longer care for themselves, and who had been abandoned by family and friends.

As a young staff psychologist I was a therapist for men like those I had treated in a large Army hospital four years earlier, and who at that time were fresh from combat. Now these men were aged and sadder.

Glancing about, I noticed a little old man at the other end of the bench, muttering to himself and stroking his dog. I had been told about Andrew and his dog by a senior social worker who had talked with him a long time ago, when he was still communicating with others. Now he sat silently, staring out into space, occasionally patting "Rex," and mumbling words of endearment. According to my informant Rex was a sheepdog which had been with Andrew for many years.

Andrew had returned from France in 1918, shattered in spirit and helpless to cope with a different world. His had been destroyed in a hail of artillery explosions, machine-gun fire, slaughtered buddies, men with their arms and legs blown off, and mud, mud, mud.

Adventures in Human Understanding

In and out of the trenches he and the other khaki-clad boys wearing flat helmets had climbed, bayoneting and being bayoneted by other young men dressed in gray who wore pot-shaped headwear. And when the victory parades celebrated the return of heroes, the hospital ships returned carrying those who had physically escaped a permanent sleep in Flanders Field, but who had never emotionally left their world of horror. So it was with Andrew.

Although he was not housed in my ward I was curious about him. He appeared not to hear me but stared at the far distance, altering his gaze only occasionally to pat his dog and utter a few kind words. "Atta boy, Rex. Good dog." So Andrew and I sat beside one another, both enjoying this quiet, beautiful scene, close together, and yet isolated beings, eons apart.

"Shell shock" it was called in those days. With some, it maimed body and with others, spirit, but let no one doubt its reality. There were thousands like Andrew, who, suffering from this malady, returned to a still partly sane world, and tried to fit in.

Nobody came to visit Andrew—no friends, no relatives, not even an acquaintance who might have known him. Now Andrew's contact with the world was only through his dog. And he had been at the hospital so long that no present staff members could even remember when he arrived.

We sat silently together for perhaps a half-hour. Although he never glanced at me, I was observing him carefully, wrinkled old face, turned-up nose, disheveled grayish-white hair and beard, he wore baggy clothes, seldom changed. Andrew sat quietly, patting Rex occasionally, but otherwise totally involved in his own thoughts.

My notes made from records in the Personnel Department showed only that he had enlisted in the Army in November, 1917, had served in the cavalry, had been transferred to the States from a hospital in France, and had been honorably discharged in December, 1918. No awards, no ribbons, no citations, he had served credibly but without distinction. His unit saw combat only as infantry, since horses then could not survive the withering slaughter of machine-gun fire.

Andrew and his Old Sheepdog

Andrew was now an ancient nobody, spending the rest of a meaningless life in a beautiful nowhere, ignored alike by staff and inmates. But he was not alone; he had his dog, Rex.

Wherever Andrew went, Rex was always at his side. To the exercise gym where all the inmates were taken each day—whether they wished to or not. To the infrequent medical check-ups. To the rose garden, where sometimes they both spent a warm afternoon. But mostly to the confines of his small and dimly lit room. There Andrew would either lie on his cot staring at the ceiling, or sit in the single wooden chair chuckling to himself while patting Rex. Andrew had placed a pad on the floor between the chair and his cot where the dog could slumber.

One morning we sat on the bench a long time. When the noon hour arrived, Andrew stirred, turned to Rex and remarked, "Come on, Boy. Time for us to go." He then painfully rose, and with bent back and bowed head shuffled his gaunt frame toward the mess hall.

I followed at a respectful distance, interested in what would take place. Andrew seated himself in a chair at the end of a small table and motioned for Rex to sit down beside him, then bit by bit he consumed the modest fare provided. Occasionally he would look down at Rex and offer the dog a morsel of food.

I had heard that when Andrew and Rex first arrived at the hospital, some of the mess hall attendants objected, insisting that this arrangement would disturb other inmates. However, apparently the matter had been long settled, since nobody was upset when Andrew was seated.

There were many other times when I joined Andrew on the lakeside bench and wondered what he was pondering when he stared so long and silently into space. Could it be that he was once again a curly-headed lad frolicking with his dog in the sunshine, shouting, "Hya, Rex. Go gettum, Boy," as "little Andy" threw a stick which Rex would fetch? Maybe he had later acquired the present Rex because the dog would remind him of his childhood, where he was once happy. Was this dog his tangible connection to that earlier time?

Adventures in Human Understanding

Or maybe his memories were of a proud father and mother admiring him as he rode his horse around the ranch. I didn't know that he had lived on a ranch. I imagined it only because he had joined the cavalry. Perhaps those were not his thoughts. Maybe he was remembering when he enlisted in the Service and was issued his first scratchy, khaki wool shirt, standard in those days ("G.I." we would have called it in World War II). Sometimes I wondered if Andrew's fond mother kept a blue flag with a silver star in her window while patiently awaiting his return from France. And where was she now, certainly long dead? With a start I returned from this world of imagination to one of reality. I knew nothing about Andrew, and I was creating in him a fantasized childhood, a real young somebody through my own imagination. Nor did I have knowledge regarding his family. The favorable images I had created may have simply been transferred from memories of my own caring parents.

A better psychological rationale to account for such a severe disability would have suggested that he came from a very abusive home, one in which beatings and verbal humiliation prevailed. And that "Andy," a sensitive child, had found he could escape the brutality only by running with his dog to hide. For a little while he could be safe, secure and with a "friend," who would never hurt him. Perhaps he later "ran" mentally from the horror of the killing fields in France into an inner hiding place, and then acquired Rex as his sole companion. How could we know what really happened in Andrew's childhood?

Therapists are supposed to acquire "insight" into the early experiences, fears, hates, loves and conflicts which may have determined later reactions to great stress and interpret this understanding to their patients. But when the patient not only fails to communicate, but doesn't even recognize the very existence of the therapist, what can one do to help?

"No man is an Iland, intire of it selfe, every man is a peece of the Continent, a part of the maine," wrote John Donne in 1623. Each of us must somehow have contact with the rest of the "Continent" of mankind. And if our "Iland" has no bridge to another being, we must build that bridge. But if we can, then we are safe.

Even when my good wife and I were weathering through hurricane George on the island of St. Thomas, there was support from other storm watchers, plus radio and television communication with the mainland. We were never alone. But when all bridges to other human "Ilands" are gone perhaps the Creator has endowed us with the where-with-all to acquire and establish contact with some external, non-self reality, such as another life form, thus making it possible for us to exist. For only when our "self" and something that is "not-self" touch each other can "conscious awareness" really take place. Andrew's contact was with Rex, the always faithful one. With Rex at his side Andrew could afford to exist.

Years later, on visiting the hospital I heard that Andrew had died. Reminiscing, I imagined him lying on his cot during those last moments. He probably reached out, patted Rex on the head and muttered, "Come on, Boy. Time for us to go." Then closing his eyes they went together to that encampment in the sky where he would meet again those buddies he left in the fields of France. Maybe an unusually kind and understanding "Commanding Officer" would also be there, one who would not object to Rex lying on the tent floor beside Andrew's cot. Each of us must have someone toward whom we can give and receive love—even if that someone is only an hallucinated old sheepdog named Rex.

Thoughts of a Therapist: Analysis and Comment

There is little action in this "story," only observations of the psychologist/writer. Andrew as a consequence of his battle trauma has become mute. Sometimes, when we have suffered more harmful impact than we can handle, we may retreat into an inner world. We are then diagnosed as "psychotic." So it was with Andrew.

He illustrates the horrors of war, which, unless we have actually experienced them, we can only imagine. Much of this discussion was the imagination of the observer. However, it is easy to let our imaginations create a rationale to explain a psychological condition—which may or may not be true.

Adventures in Human Understanding

Several quite different childhood scripts could account for Andrew's irrational behavior. These behaviors are consistent within themselves. They are presented from an attempt by the observing psychologist to insert himself into Andrew and consider how he would have reacted if he had suffered Andrew's battlefield trauma.

Putting one's self into "another person's skin" and co-experiencing it is called "resonance," an extreme form of "empathy." Even the final "death" of Andrew is told as how an observing therapist might have imagined it.

The lessons here: 1. The horrors of war, 2. The drastic retreats from real living forced on many of its victims, and 3. The recognition that love of "something" or "someone" "outside of one's own self" is necessary for psychological survival.

An hallucination is not felt as one's "thought," hence, coming from within one's own "self." It is experienced like in a dream, as an outside object, a perception. Andrew created the hallucination of "Rex" because there was nobody left in his real world to whom he could relate.

Chapter 11

Buddies

"I tell you, kids have no sense of responsibility today."

Lars Olson was holding forth on a favorite topic to his buddy, Jim Malone. Both were residents at the Veteran's Retirement facility in south Oregon. Older brick buildings and newer replacements mingled, spreading over spacious green lawns punctuated by many trees.

The rainy season would soon descend onto this refuge for veterans, who were no longer able to remain self-supporting, and the "old boys" were taking advantage of the bright October sunshine. Some strolled the walkways. Others stretched out on the park benches which dotted the grounds. Lars and Jim were seated on the same wooden bench to which they laid claim when, weather permitting, they could just relax and "shoot the breeze."

Lars, with his snow-white hair and beard, presented a regal appearance in spite of his stooped shoulders. He would often reminisce about the past, but could easily forget what he had just said and then might repeat himself.

Jim, whose light brown hair was beginning to be streaked with gray, tended to listen more, but when he talked, his comments had a positive ring.

"Yeah, I know. The kids today don't volunteer for unpleasant duties, like we did when I enlisted for Vietnam. They do pot and crack too. But we used to get drunk on beer, didn't you?"

Lars retreated slightly. "Well, we did get rotgut from the bootleggers when I was in the National Guard. But we didn't drive cars like mad and cause all the wrecks they have today."

Adventures in Human Understanding

Lars liked to open an argument, but when confronted he withdrew more quickly.

"Of course you didn't," countered Jim. "The jalopies you had then couldn't go over 50 miles an hour."

So it went throughout the afternoon.

Lars was the bookish type. He would sit for hours in the reading room, eyes glued to a good Western, rarely mingling with the other inmates. He had been a resident of the facility a long time but had made no close friends before Jim arrived. Other residents shied away when they saw him in one of his "blacking-out" spells.

He would sit with his eyes closed, completely self-absorbed. During these "blackouts" Lars didn't really become unconscious. He would just fade into a private world of his past. Jim had learnt not to interrupt him because in a minute or two he would snap out of it. Occasionally Lars would break out in spells of hysterical crying.

Jim was a newcomer. When he arrived three months ago, he and Lars immediately hit it off. You'd think they had been lifelong pals. Now they ate meals together and spent much of the time talking, walking, and playing games, mostly checkers or horseshoes. Lars's "blacking-out" spells were fewer, and he rarely had any hysterical weeping.

At checkers, Lars was generally the winner, but he couldn't match Jim in horseshoes. Jim had been an athlete and liked games of physical skill. Still, there was some magic between them.

Like most old soldiers, sooner or later memories of their time in uniform would emerge. Today it was Lars's turn. Staring at the blue sky with a blank look on his wrinkled features, he once more relived another time and place.

"I was in the 116th Cavalry, Idaho National Guard. Enlisted when I was eighteen. Ended up as a sergeant. Before the war we'd go to summer camp—drill and stand guard mount. That's where you line up your horses, draw sabres and parade in front of the reviewing stand. Since I came from a ranch near Pocatello, and had competed in local rodeos, the horse cavalry was just what I wanted. When we were mustered into the regular army they sent us to the Armored School at Fort Bragg. Horses were out, and we learned to handle tanks.

"I had a close buddy, Tom. We had enlisted together. He was a real neat guy. We would shoot the bull together for hours. His girlfriend lived in Rupert, and they were going to get married when the war was over."

There was a long pause. Lars began to sweat profusely. His face looked like the middle of a thunderstorm, and his legs shook violently. Something drastic within was happening. Jim, who had seen this reaction before, moved instinctively closer and put his arm around Lars's shoulder.

"Tom and I were in a Sherman tank together in '44. They dropped us at the Anzio Beachhead. For the first few days nothing much happened. Spent most of the time unloading supplies. Then all hell broke loose. The Panzers started coming."

Suddenly Lars was no longer in the veterans' home. For the moment he was back on the beaches of Italy. Its horror was here and now as he screamed, "Look out, Tom! Here comes another 88."

Lars collapsed in a torrent of tears and dived off the bench. Lying on the ground he beat the grass helplessly with both arms.

"Oh my God. Oh my God. He's on fire. Get out, Tom. I can't move." He returned to the present.

"Why couldn't I have helped him? Why didn't I pull him out and beat down the flames? I'm no damned good, a damn poor soldier."

Jim moved closer on the park bench. In another minute the wailing subsided.

"I was lucky. Jumped out and landed on my back. Tom didn't make it—that is, he got out of the tank, but there was fire all over him. God, I couldn't get to him. I heard him scream while he was burning up, then he was gone. Can still hear that scream."

Lars buried his face on Jim's shoulder. The rainstorm of tears continued. Between hysterical sobs, Lars relived once again the same story which his buddy had already heard before. Jim knew it couldn't be stopped. Each time it had to wear itself out. Lars took a rumpled handkerchief from his pants pocket and wiped his face.

"Got a shell fragment in my arm," he reiterated, pointing to a scar just above the tattoo of crossed sabres on his biceps.

"I went loco. They called it 'combat fatigue.' In the hospital I'd wake up screaming. They sent me to a hospital in Florida, and a shrink there straightened me out—I guess. Then I was discharged."

The sobbing quieted down. Lars slumped into a helpless puddle. Jim knew the worst was over.

"Tom was the best buddy I ever had. Haven't found one like him since. Don't care for most of the guys here."

Jim sat quietly, but every time Lars dived into his terrible memories, they seemed to pull out similar ones in Jim. He, too, had to get them off his chest. Each time they shared experiences in the horrors of combat it cemented further their common bond. When Jim opened up, his revelations were always much calmer, and he never lost his rational sense of present time and place.

"That sure was hell, Lars. I wasn't in combat as long as you were. It was a different kind of battle in the jungles of Vietnam. I, too, had my buddies shot down, but I was never as close to any other guy as you were to Tom.

"Soon after we got to 'Nam they sent us out on patrols. At night you couldn't see a damned thing. You never knew whether you were firing at our goops or their goops. It really got me seeing women and little kids in the villages slaughtered. The goops would blast the huts with mortar shells when they thought we were hiding inside. Then when the 'Nam family ran out they'd be mowed down. I couldn't tell whether it was our guys or theirs who did most of the killing. They were blasted in a rain of mortar shells from both the enemy and our own troops."

Jim paused a moment as if he needed to get his second wind before proceeding to face his worst horror again.

"One night we were close to Da Nang. I never saw that cord across the trail. The damn land mine blew off my leg." He ruefully pointed to his stump on the left side.

"The VA made a metal leg for me, but the stupid government docs messed it up. I kept complaining. Never got anything back but a form letter promising to look into the matter. Even wrote Senator Murray, who also promised to get some action. Still nothing happened. The artificial leg never fitted, so most of the time I'd just rather use my crutch." Jim reached over and retrieved a beaten-up wooden crutch from the other side of the bench.

Lars was beginning to recover. He wanted to change the subject—even though he couldn't quite blot out the image of Tom on fire.

"What did ya do before you got in the Army?"

"I was in college for two years before enlisting. Thought it was my duty to join up. You know, wave the flag thing. Played basketball with the Oregon Ducks. Damn good too. Thought I had a real chance at the professionals. I wanted to be like Chamberlain and those other guys. They sure make a lot of money. After 'Nam, no chance."

This tripped off a more benign memory in Lars, who was by now almost out of his ugly spell.

"I had a brother-in-law who married my sister. They lived in Corvallis. He was a big better on basketball games. Did you ever play the Beavers at Oregon State? I used to visit him, and he'd take me to the games."

"When was that?" broke in Jim, also wishing to change the painful topic.

Adventures in Human Understanding

"In the winter of '40 I think."

Jim cupped his hands and pretended he was throwing the ball at a basket.

"We sure did. Won too."

"I was there in '40. Might have seen you play."

"Well, I'll be damned," replied Jim with a smile on his face. "It's a small world."

The tension from combat stories eased off. Talk shifted to basketball tournaments. They had shared their most painful moments and felt closer to one another.

"Let's play checkers," suggested Lars.

Jim knew he'd probably be beaten. But he felt so pleased about their moment of common recognition that he didn't care. So off they went together to the game room.

It was bright sunshine the next day when, sitting on their favorite bench, the conversation turned toward more personal matters. Jim led off.

"Whatcha do after you left the Army?"

"Not much. Tried working in a service station. I was fired."

Jim broke in. "How come?"

"I'd get angry, blow my top, cuss somebody out, and then I'd lose my job. Never got over that loss of Tom. Finally I applied for admission here. Been here 20 years. Kind of a dull life, but it's O.K. They feed you well."

Jim, sensing he was getting into paydirt area, started some more personal questions.

"Did you ever get married?"

"Could have, once. A real nice gal, but I didn't follow through. I guess I'm not the marrying type. Even tried to find her, but the family had moved away. Years later, after I knew I'd probably always be a bachelor, I used to wonder what it would be like to have a son, you know, like you could take fishing and teach him how to read."

"How about you?"

Jim stretched his 6'4" frame out where it was more comfortable on the bench. Because of the one leg, you'd never guess he was that tall.

"Yeah! Did get married once. We never had any kids. She got tired of me. Took off with some guy. Just as well, I guess. Women don't want a man with one leg."

Lars was silent, and Jim just waited. He noticed that Lars had his eyes closed and was in one of his reverie periods. He'd make little motions as if he were thinking and playing something out.

Lars had indeed left the present scene. This talk about girls had started something. He was back in the days before the war, back in the 116th Cavalry, and he was 19 years old.

Lars's military unit had been transported from Pocatello to the summer encampment of the Idaho National Guard at Fort Boise. The 230 miles of bouncing in an army truck was tiresome, and they still had to put up the tents before they could turn-in. Lars had slept like a log and was startled by the bugle call at reveille the next morning. He wasn't accustomed to getting up at 5:00 a.m. Just time to make up your bunk then stand inspection (not a single crease permitted). No time to snooze. The whole troop was rousted out for breakfast, then to an "orientation" talk. This proved to be more interesting.

"Listen, you guys," said the gray-haired chicken colonel, who was chief medical officer. "If you don't take precautions when you screw a girl you can get the clap, or even syphilis. And if you

Adventures in Human Understanding

knock her up, man, you've got trouble. Go to the dispensary and get some condoms. Carry them with you whenever you go to town—even if you don't intend to use them."

Lars felt somewhat intimidated by the lecture from this high-ranking officer, but he did as he was told—and then forgot the matter. Actually, he was shocked at such frank talk. Words like that were not allowed on the ranch by his church-going parents. Of course, there had been a lot of "sneak-talk" in the grade school, mostly just talk.

That evening the boys were shooting the bull just before taps in an eight-man tent. Corporal Bart Thomas was describing his most recent conquest. He was older than the rest of the troop—had his black hair slicked down, like Rudolph Valentino's in the movies.

"I sure did score with her."

Boise girls were more modest in those days. But still it was expected that every guy would try. There was quite a bit of bragging about "scores," many more claimed than games played.

Corporal Thomas continued: "There are different steps in making a girl. You hafta time it right. First, don't be in a hurry. Girls like plenty of romancing. You know, nice talk and a few kisses. After a while they get warmed up. Then you go to the second step. You increase the number of kisses and hold them longer. You start stroking their cheeks, neck and arms. You can tell by their breathing when they're turned on." Lars was all ears. This was important know-how.

The fellows now were sitting on their bunks in rapt attention. Many of them were still in their early teens—the captain lied about their age. With no war in sight they had signed up because they couldn't get a job. The youngest ones were often away from home for the first time.

"The next step is to stroke her legs and breasts, but don't be in a hurry yet. Then when she's breathing real heavy and kissing back at you passionately you put your hand down between her legs.

Once you touch her there, and she doesn't object, you know she's ready."

Lars was very impressed with Corporal Thomas, even more than with the medical officer. It's not often you get such advice from an expert. He could hardly wait to try out his newly learned skill. He even wrote down the basic steps in a notebook and stuck it in his duffle bag.

The summer before, he had met a slender, black-haired teenager who fired his imagination. They had gone swimming twice at the "natatorium," but a hamburger and a milkshake afterwards was all that happened before he had taken her home. Lars was too shy to go further. He figured then she'd say, "No," and he didn't want to lose her. But now a year older, and reinforced with all this "man-talk" about what turns girls on, he was challenged to a more aggressive try.

That Sunday afternoon he and Rosie had another date. They met at the Idanha Hotel, went to the matinee at the Pinney, and then took the old trolley which rattled up Warm Springs Avenue to the natatorium. It was fun getting bumped against her occasionally. When he first saw Rosie in her bathing suit at the pool, even more pleasurable possibilities suggested themselves. She was sure "stacked."

Rosie knew how to smooth a male bird's feathers. "I hear you're an expert swimmer."

Lars, wearing his new blue swimsuit with the Red Cross lifeguard insignia in the middle, stretched himself a bit taller. He then did several one-and-a-half spins from the high board. Rosie was impressed.

"Gee. You sure are strong, Lars."

It was early evening when they took the trolley back down town and strolled through the Capitol grounds. Big dome, statues, tall oak trees, expansive lawns. They were soon reclining in the midst of a clump of flowering bushes. The evening shadows left little light. Since the State personnel had left for the day, there was nobody around.

Lars had kissed her once the year before and maybe two or three times recently—rather modest little pecks. But this time, when he kissed her, she put her arms around him and pulled him close. One kiss led to another, and soon he found himself pulling his pants down and her dress up. Somehow he forgot all about the important "steps" which Corporal Thomas had maintained were a necessary prerequisite. In fact he was absolutely overwhelmed as Rosie took complete charge of the situation.

The ending of this episode was fore-ordained when Adam first met Eve. Time stood still. Bliss reigned.

Putting on their clothes, they lay together for about an hour, while Rosie kissed and patted him. Finally in a state of confusion Lars confided, "You're wonderful, Rosie. I love you," not knowing whether he meant it, or even what it was to be in love. However, he did sense a very relaxed glow, something he'd never experienced before. He must be in love with her.

Neither of them had any awareness of time as, holding hands, they slowly strolled back to her home. A quick kiss on the porch. Lars scurried off when her mother anxiously turned on the porch light.

It was dark. On his way back to the camp Lars had very mixed feelings. He was still musing when he arrived at the gates to the Fort.

"Halt! Who goes there?" shouted the sentry.

In those days that seemed unnecessary. World War I was a long time ago. And the possibility of a World War II never occurred to anybody. No enemy would be attacking Fort Boise. However, Lars gave the expected response,

"None of your damn business."

"Pass on, soldier," grumbled the shivering guard, hoping his relief would not be late.

Lars continued pondering while laying on his cot. He was so immersed in his daydream that he was quite oblivious of the chorus of snores in the tent. Now he had "scored." He was a man. And he had a right to brag about his conquest at the evening bullfest. But somehow it didn't seem right. She was a nice girl, and the promptings he got from her were not all lusty ones. At any rate he said nothing about "the score" that night, or afterward. However, when unlacing his leggings and removing his pants that night he discovered in his pocket the unused pack of condoms.

"Oh! I sure forgot. Probably nothing to worry about."

During the hot middle-of-July afternoons, when they were permitted to rest in the shade of the tents, most of the guys shed their leggings, unbuttoned their scratchy, khaki shirts and took naps. Lars, however, couldn't get Rosie off his mind.

The 143rd Artillery Battalion with their 75 mm guns was practicing marksmanship in the foothills behind Fort Boise. For awhile it was fun to watch the spouts of dust where the shells hit and then count seconds before you heard the boom. But neither those explosions, nor the snores of his buddies in B Troop, could intrude on Lars's reveries while he relived over and over again those delicious moments of ecstasy on the Capitol grounds. "Wow! Rosie was sure something."

The two-week encampment was over. They packed all their gear, loaded the trucks and returned home. Military duty now was only one evening a week until next year.

Six weeks later, while Lars was pitching hay in the barn, his mother called out to him, "Lars, there's some girl wanting to talk to you on the phone. Long distance, I think."

Mrs. Olson went into the kitchen and closed the door. Although his mother was a prim, church-going, "Victorian" matron, she never interfered with the dates of her sons nor inquired what she knew was none of her business.

Adventures in Human Understanding

Lars lifted the earphone to his ear. It was Rosie's voice. "Lars. You and I are going to have a baby."

He nearly fell off the stool, which stood by the wall where the phone was bolted.

"Uh! What'd you say?"

"A baby. We're going to have a baby."

Lars was absolutely dumbfounded. Nothing like this had ever occurred to him. He was completely incapable of coping with such an announcement. He stammered a few words.

"That can't be. Are you sure it isn't a mistake?"

Rosie, a bright little girl who could always manage a snappy comeback, replied, "It was a mistake, alright. But what are you going to do about it?"

"What am I going to do about it? I can't do anything about it."

"I know. You've done too much already, but what are you going to do about it *now*?"

Never in his life had Lars been called upon to deal with such a situation. His head was in a whirl as he searched for some solution.

"Can't you do something? You know, there are doctors in Boise, aren't there?"

"Lars! Shame on you. That would be a mortal sin. I could never go to confession—let alone tell the priest about it."

Lars felt cornered. He was absolutely speechless. "Well-uh. I'm not the marrying type. Mother told me I shouldn't even think of marriage until I was at least 25. She said, 'How're you going to support a wife until you complete your education and get a job? You haven't got a nickel to your name.'"

There was a click and no more Rosie. She had slammed the phone down on the hook. Lars thought a long time. He didn't want to get married, just couldn't get married right now and really couldn't have said anything different. But he didn't feel right about blaming his mother for the problem. The gnawing feeling of guilt didn't go away.

During the next two months he tried to call Rosie. The line always seemed to be busy. He kept thinking. Maybe she had just missed her period, and it was a false alarm. Surely if she was pregnant she would contact him again. This line of thought continued for many months before he decided maybe he'd better settle the matter once and for all.

Getting his old jalopy in good running shape (that is for a 1936 Model A) he set out one weekend for Boise. 1225 4th Avenue. He knocked at the door. A pleasant little gray-haired lady carrying a broom answered.

"Rosie? No they moved away a month ago. We bought their house. They went West somewhere. Didn't leave a forwarding address. No idea where you can get in touch with them."

Lars returned to the ranch, mulling his mind over many competing ideas.

"If she had been pregnant, and he was the father, wouldn't she surely have called him again? Still, she was a spunky little gal. Proud. Had a mind of her own. Maybe she just gave up on him." That didn't make much sense to Lars. "She probably was just late with her period. There was no baby, and he needn't worry about it. Yes, that was the answer."

Years passed. The whole matter faded from Lars' mind. War came to America. His outfit was mobilized, and other problems completely occupied his attention.

A backfire from the exhaust of a truck bringing supplies to the VA facility suddenly exploded, jarring Lars out of his reverie.

Adventures in Human Understanding

"We were talking—? Oh yes, what happened before the War."

It was several days later before Lars and Jim found time to get together. A rock band was giving the veterans an afternoon concert. They were very loud, and conversation was impossible. The next day there was a contest, best answers in a quiz game. Then visitors' day. The facility was crowded with family members and friends. It rained for three days. Too chilly to go outside. Lars spent time in the library, and Jim played dartboard in the game room with some of the other residents.

The next Friday the clouds thinned, and the sun seemed almost ready to break through. The two agreed to meet at the same park bench. There was an air of expectancy. Something intangible about Jim made Lars want to find out more about his friend's past. He offered an opening.

"I guess you've heard what there is to know about me. What did you do before the war?"

Unlike Lars, Jim seemed quite alert when he was reminiscing.

"We moved to Eugene when I was very little. My uncle had a 'mom-and-pop' store. He took us in. We Irish stick together. My father had been killed. Drowning accident, I understand. Mother never wanted to talk about it. I believe he was trying to save a high school buddy when they went boating on the Snake river. He was never found. She must have been quite upset. She never said a bad word about him. I think she was always in love with him. It made me feel good to know she loved and admired him. You can be proud when your Dad is that kind of guy. Wished I had known him. We could have played games, baseball, volleyball, and gone swimming together. At the ball games in high school all the other fellows came with their dads. A boy sure misses not having a father."

Lars momentarily felt the cold gust of wind as a cloud passed over the sun.

"You never had a father?"

"Well, I did have a father for awhile. My Mom married Kevin Malone when I was still a baby. I think she was tired of living alone. He adopted me, but I never thought of him as my Dad. On the road all the time. He was a traveling salesman for some agricultural machines firm. Wasn't mean, just aloof. He died of heart failure when I was five. Mother never married again.

"She was a hard worker. Never complained about anything. Took over the job of cook and waitress at the lunch counter in my uncle's store."

Lars sensed a growing interest. Part of him wanted to ask more about her. Part of him didn't—and another part felt it was getting too chilly outside. It would be warm back in his room or in the library. Another two minutes of "blacking out" as Jim just sat quietly contemplating the gold leaves on the foliage above.

Finally Lars jerked back alert.

"What was your mom like, Jim?" he asked.

"Oh, she was a spitfire. Had a real Irish temper and was proud. When she said something, she meant it. Her hair was darker than mine. They used to joke about my being a towhead when I was little. I never figured how she could be so short, about 5 foot, when I got to be 6'4". Mom loved swimming. Bought a season ticket to the municipal pool, and we'd go there together. She was a good swimmer. Taught me the crawl."

Wheels began to grind in Lars's head. He would alternately seem to be absorbed in calculating, wincing, stretching his gaunt frame, then wiggling his shoulders back and forth, like he both did and didn't want to do something.

"Jim, you said your family moved to Eugene when you were a baby. When was that?"

"I don't know exactly. I learned about it later when I went to school and they asked my birth date and place. I think it was early in the depression days."

Adventures in Human Understanding

Lars was beginning to feel increasingly uneasy. Several questions kept popping up in his mind. He felt he ought to ask them, but he resisted for quite a while.

"Jim, how old are you?"

"I'll be 66 come next April. How old are you?"

Without thinking, Lars replied, "I'm 86."

Lars felt a pressure that was getting stronger with each passing moment. Like it was about to burst the dam. He didn't want it to, but he did want it to. He knew, though, he had to ask the next one.

"You said your family moved to Eugene when you were only a baby. Where was that from?"

"I guess I forgot to mention. I was born in Boise, Idaho. Beautiful town. Ever been there?"

Lars sat straight up on the bench, stared ahead, and went into another blanking state. This time it was almost five minutes before he came out of it. And when he did it was like emerging from a foggy cloud into warm sunlight. He was taking big breaths and appeared to be excited.

"Anything wrong?" asked Jim.

"No. Nothing at all. Nothing at all."

Gradually the stiffness went out of Lars. He seemed to melt almost comfortably into the bench before he stood up and stretched. Jim wondered what he was smiling about. "How about going for supper?"

"Good idea."

Jim reached for his cane, while Lars took his arm on the other side, ostensibly to support his one-footed comrade. An equally good reason would be that when holding Jim's arm Lars never went into one of his "blacking-outs."

The sun was low over the western mountains when Lars commented, "The sun's about to set. We don't have much time."

But Jim, who was more optimistic, replied, "Look. There's quite a bit of daylight left. If we hurry eating we'll still have time for several horseshoe games. I like playing games with you."

"I like playing games with you, too," replied Lars.

Then he added something strange. "I wish we could have played games together—a long time ago." He reached over and patted the younger fellow on the shoulder. For a moment this comment puzzled Jim. But he put it aside. The sun was still shining above the western mountains, and there would be a little more daylight before the shadows of night took over. Slowly the two "buddies," arm in arm, hobbled across the green lawn to have supper, then play games—together.

Thoughts of a Therapist: Analysis and Comment

Lars Olson and Jim Malone, two old soldiers in a Veterans' Home, become close friends. Although from different generations, World War II and the Vietnam War, they are instinctively drawn together.

Lars, the elder, complains of irresponsibility in today's adolescents, not realizing that when he was young he manifested the same carefree lack of responsibility himself.

As is common with veterans, they compare military experiences; both of them underwent severe and disabling traumas. Each describes his own in the language and customs of his generation. Increasingly, they discover more common ground.

Lars is given to reminiscing, which trips off the reliving of a traumatic event involving the death by fire of a close buddy. During these "blacking-out" periods he often loses contact with the present and re-experiences the event as if it were happening in the here-and-now.

Adventures in Human Understanding

Jim, who has lost a leg, is more calm and reconciled. His disability is not diagnosed as "psychiatric."

In one of his "blacking-out" reminiscences, Lars returns to his teenage service in the National Guard. Here he, a farm boy, "learns" about sex from a medical officer and from an older soldier who is an "expert" with women. He determines to prove his manhood by "scoring" with a teenage girlfriend.

He is successful, but with the active acquiescence of his young partner. When she informs him later that she is pregnant, he is completely unable to face the challenge and take responsibility.

They lose track of each other. His cavalry outfit is sent to the battlefields in Europe. Later, he regrets never finding out whether or not he is a father. He wished that he could have had a son.

As they grow older and more mature, people often regret the immature behaviors of their youth—if they have not forgotten them through repression or normal loss of memory.

Jim confides in Lars his lifelong wish to have had a father. And, as they are drawn together, Lars becomes increasingly aware that Jim is probably his own son. In the end Lars, but not Jim, realizes this as fact. Lars keeps this understanding to himself.

There are many little innuendos and symbolic meanings transmitted between the two. Lars, aware of his own approaching death (age 86)—but unconsciously, notes that *"the sun is about to set,"* and *"We don't have much time."*

Jim, a robust 66, (not recognizing the underlying meaning of that remark) optimistically responds. "There's quite a bit of daylight left."

The two "buddies" leave for the mess hall, arm in arm, as they "celebrate" their newly uncovered father-son relationship, one with conscious knowledge, the other (who has also "received" the good news) unconsciously. They will increasingly enjoy "playing games" together.

Chapter 12

Dao-Tsai and the White Marble Image

Many centuries ago during the reign of the Emperor Hammu, there lived in a village in the highlands west of Hakone a young man of serious mind. Hoping to become mature and revered as a man of wisdom, he journeyed to Nara and sought counsel of the great Buddha.

"Oh Mighty One," he prayed, "how can I learn The Way which leads to the portals of heaven? My father, learned teacher that he was, instructed me in many things. He showed me how to chart the courses of the moon and stars as they circle the earth, where wend the birds in their southward flight at each falling of the leaves, and how to ward off the monsters of evil who inflict the fever sickness on the careless traveler. He taught me virtue and the manly arts of war. He instilled in me a reverence for my ancestors, for the gods and for service to the emperor. In the great university at Heiankyo I learned to read the ancient parchments, to sing the songs of the classic poets, and to practice the ceremonies and courtesies which have ever marked our people. All these things I did learn and yet—and yet I would achieve the blissful life, the serenity of existence and the peace of greatness before I, too, depart for the realms of my forefathers. How, oh Great One, is this to be found? Can you tell me The Way?"

No sound came from the Buddha who had sat in majestic contemplation for many, many years. The frailties, the follies of thousands of men had passed before his eyes. Yes, and also the few, the very few, who had somehow managed to find The Way before the god of darkness had struck them down.

Adventures in Human Understanding

No word passes from his lips, but for those whose hearts are ready and whose minds are open the Buddha speaks directly to the inner recesses of the soul.

"My Son, The Way is long. It is not to be attained except by him who searches well and seeks diligently to achieve. The quest is not for the feeble resolve, those who are impatient, nor those who are unwilling to sacrifice."

Dao fought back many misgivings as his needs on the one hand and doubts of his worthiness on the other struggled for ascendancy.

"Oh Great Buddha, I am but small. I have never been called to high post by the emperor. I have vanquished no enemies in battle. Nor have I inscribed song or verse that will be left to posterity. But I have a stout heart; I am not afraid, and I will seek The Way even though it takes a lifetime. Tell me the path that I may set my steps thereon and reach the goal of what man's striving is all about. Point The Way to me, and I will travel there, though it takes many moons."

The voice of the Buddha was soft but firm. "Young and Eager One, I cannot tell you The Way. Each man must discover it for himself. There is but one who knows The Way, and you must find him, for only he can tell you of its course."

Dao was shaken. Was it possible that the Buddha knew not The Way, that some other being, god or man, possessed alone this knowledge? And where was such a being to be found? He felt certain in his heart that if he prayed earnestly, and if he searched assiduously, the Buddha would reveal to him that which his entire self craved to understand. He had journeyed a long distance, and now he was instructed to begin a new search for one of whose nature and whereabouts he knew not.

"But how shall I recognize this being who has knowledge of The Way? Where is he to be found? And when will I meet him?"

There was a long pause as if the Buddha were weighing whether or not he would speak again.

"I do not know where you will find him, nor when you will meet him. Many men never see him. And many others spend wasted lives very close to him yet never recognize his features. I wish you good fortune in your quest, but all the rest is up to you."

In anguish lest the Buddha speak no further, Dao cried out, "But Great One, can you at least instruct me in one tiny step, one slight move that may turn my journey in his direction? If you do not help me then I am lost, for I have neither the wit nor skill even to begin this search."

With solemn tones the words of the Buddha engraved themselves on the young man's mind.

"In the far north, at the uttermost reaches of our island where the sky and the majestic ocean sweep to a meeting beyond the eyes of man, there is a stone. It is atop a cliff of jagged rock which juts into the foamy brine. And it is white; pure white marble. Hidden under its polished surface lies the image of him whom you seek. The journey will be long and dangerous as you must pass through the lands of the Ainu, and they have sworn death to all strangers.

"However, if you can find the stone and release this image from its prisoning embrace you may recognize the features of him who knows The Way. And if from this image you learn his identity you will be able to reach the object of your quest."

The Buddha was silent and seemed not to hear the pleadings of the young man for more instruction. Dao's heart beat with great dread since he did not comprehend how to release the "Knower-of-The-Way" from the white stone. He sought with all his concentration to contact once again the mind of the Buddha.

The sun had set, and the grayness of nightfall crept over the land. Dark was the moon, and a cold wind whistled through the great shrine which housed the Buddha. Dao shivered and, thinking of the warm hearth in his house, was tempted to leave. But unless he could have assurance that he would be able to release the Knowing One from his marble shroud he knew that he must fail. Dao sank in self-contemplation. Through his innermost heart he

Adventures in Human Understanding

beseeched the Buddha to speak again and reveal to him how he could penetrate the marble stone.

As if from a million miles away a small, still voice, soft indeed but like a resonant whisper, stirred his being.

"My Son, you must patiently chip away the stone, tiny piece by tiny piece. But do not lose courage. It is the heart, and not the mind, that will prevail. Neither by logic nor by skill can the right bits be struck away. You cannot plan this sculpture. Let happen what will. At the same time keep in mind the highest purposes; if you ever strive to do that which you think right to do, and if you can to your own best nature remain faithful, then the Great Being of the Universe will guide your hand. The chips from the marble will fall true. He-Who-Knows-The-Way will be released, and you will recognize him. I am not sure you have the patience to continue your efforts until this final goal is reached. Few do, and it will take a very long time. I speak no more."

The full darkness of night now enveloped the massive figure of the Buddha. Dao could no longer see his face. Only the great feet, folded on the pedestal, were still visible.

Through the raging sleet, Dao retraced his steps back to his little cottage in the hills, a solitary figure bracing his shoulders against the demons of the wind. No other man or beast was to be seen, since this was a night where all living things closed their doors and remained in their shelters. But as Dao slowly trudged toward his home, the words of the Buddha passed through his mind over and over, and he resolved to undertake the journey to the North.

It was several days later when, with provisions, a blanket on his back, and a stout cane in his hand, Dao set out on the path which led through the hills, along the seashore and up toward the north land.

Soon he had left the highlands and reached the road at Tokaido, which was facing the eastern ocean. Then he began the long journey north, stopping each night at a way station: Kambara, Yoshiwara, Hara, Namazu, Mishima, Hakone, Odawara, Oiso, Hiratsuka and so on, day after tiring day slowly making his way through the civilized lands and on up into the regions of the Ainu. Here he often traveled at night and slept in the forest during the daylight so as not to attract their attention.

It was late in the year, and only the laurel leaves covered the forest ground. Occasionally a small deer, startled from its hiding place midst the bushes, darted across Dao's way. As he approached the northern regions the snow began to fall. After many days he reached the point where raged the great ocean. He could hardly see a foot ahead, so blinding was the driving sleet. A sheer cliff reared its jagged head above the churning foam below, but it was covered with snow, gleaming white snow.

Dao wandered many times over the top of this point searching for a white marble stone, perhaps buried under a mantle of wet white snow. Probing with his staff and beating with the broom he had cut from a holly tree, he sought patiently but with little success for that which the Buddha had predicted would be here. Icicles formed in his hair, and his fingers began to feel like frozen claws. The marble stone was nowhere to be seen, and he had covered every inch of the plateau which topped the cliff. Exhausted, despairing, stumbling every other step, he found a small crevice into which he could huddle his body. He had failed in his quest, but at least he had a small bit of shelter from the cold and the driving snow.

Dao did not know how long he slept, but as his eyes opened he gazed out on a scene which was wildly beautiful, terrifyingly beautiful. The sun shone brightly on the rocky knoll and revealed that it was covered with deep snow whose thickness reached to the top of his knees.

The deep azure of the sky and that of the placid sea struggled in blazing competition to capture the eye of the beholder. Dao was alone, thrust mediate between heaven and earth. As he tried to move his stiff limbs a slight recollection penetrated the murky veil of his lingering drowsiness. What was it that drummed away at his consciousness? Was it the voice of the Buddha, or was it some sixth sense, some vestige of a primitive wisdom which perhaps had come from his ancestors? It was as if he had read words somewhere that said, "The real is underneath; it is always underneath."

Adventures in Human Understanding

"What is real? What is underneath? Real-underneath. Real-underneath. Real-underneath." Round and round in Dao's mind coursed these phrases like the mournful cry of a great owl.

A dawning light began to appear in his thoughts. Dao sprang to his feet. "That which I seek is real, and it lies underneath. Underneath what? I have missed it because I sought only what was apparent, I did not look underneath. Oh yes, at the very top there was a small pile of stones. I brushed away the snow, but none of them as made of white marble. Perhaps—maybe?"

Dao rushed to the summit and began digging furiously in the deep snow, clawing with his freezing fingers at the icy coldness. One small piece of rock, another, another, another. Then a tiny glimmer of white, which somehow looked different than the snow around it. With his cane he pried, breaking off its end. Finally there tumbled into view a large smooth white stone shaped like the stump of a log. Dao was barely able to move it, but with the remaining stub of his cane he could roll it a few feet. By clearing away the snow in front, then pushing it from behind, he moved it some distance before nightfall.

The ancient scrolls on which were inscribed this story are damaged at this point. Many of them have been lost in the centuries of passing time, but enough remain to tell us that Dao managed to get his stone to the south through the help of a peasant with an ox cart. Ultimately he reached the safety of his house. There he placed the stone in his garden and began chipping away. It was indeed solid, and his tools were crude, for only with the greatest of effort and perseverance did even a single small chip break off. It is said that he toiled from sun-up to sundown, day after day, but that very little change appeared in the stone.

Many winters came and went. Dao never ceased his labors, but new demands made urgent press on his time and energy. The daughter of a merchant passing by had seen him patiently chipping at the stone and stopped to inquire the nature of his work. She was fair of face and gentle of heart, and she was impressed by the steadfast purpose of this young man in pursuit of the virtuous Way. She sensed his need for companionship, for encouragement, for affection and she lingered by his side speaking goodly words

Dao-Tsai and the White Marble Image

of praise until she caught his eye. In a few days she agreed to become his wife and share the humble cottage.

Soon another mouth to feed arrived, a small but hungry mouth, and there was little time to work upon the marble stone. Yet Dao never relinquished his goal. His need to find The Way remained ever uppermost in his thoughts.

In the hope that it could be found through the wisdom of the past, Dao searched the scrolls left by the poets of the old kingdom. Painstakingly he read through the great history books, the Kojiki and the Nihon Shoki. Although he never found in them The Way he became increasingly learned and was so recognized by others. Dao had arrived at the middle age of life and could support his family modestly through tuitions paid by the more wealthy lords of the region whose sons were sent for instruction in the writings of the ancient wise ones.

Many tens of years passed. Dao's children, those that lived, became artists, warriors or servants of the emperor and began raising families of their own. Dao's long black hair was tinged with gray, and his faithful wife still toiled ever by his side. His garden was neatly fashioned with stone lanterns, cherry trees, at the center of which was a pond filled with golden carp. A miniature arching bridge passed from the pond's edge to a small island in it.

After a hard day of instructing those young ones who resisted learning the wisdom of the past, and after he had spent an hour or two chipping away at his marble stone, Dao would stroll over the little bridge onto the island and rest his weary bones by the water's edge, musing over the fierce competition of the golden carp for the bread crumbs he tossed them.

Life was not unpleasant, but although he had searched the great poems of the past, and had carved patiently for thousands of hours at his marble stone, neither The Way nor the identity of him who knew it had yet been revealed.

Dao decided to journey once more to Nara and pray again to the great Buddha of Daibutsu. Telling his students they must await his return, and bidding his wife goodbye, he set out, cane in hand. The

Adventures in Human Understanding

land was in much turmoil as the followers of the Shogun and those who held allegiance to the emperor were warring with each other. Bands of soldiers roamed the countryside, seizing food and animals from the peasants. No one's life was safe. It was with sadness in her heart that his wife said farewell, for she knew not whether he would return safely.

Dao, now in the September of his life, found the path more hard of foot than when he had traversed it in the days of his youth. He was quite exhausted when he reached the feet of the great Buddha. Wrapping a cloak about his body he huddled nearby and slept a few hours before sunset. The shadows of evening, broken but little by the oil lamps, half revealed and half concealed the face of the Buddha as he began his prayers.

"Oh Great One, many winters ago I came to you seeking to find The Way of the true existence. You told me that only one being knew it, and that I must find him. You instructed me to go to the farthest reaches of the north and locate a marble stone. Within that stone would lie the image of him whom I would seek. That I did. I found the stone and brought it back to my cottage, and for these many years I have chipped away at it. You told me that the search would be long, and that I must be patient. I resolved with my whole heart never to forsake this quest. Yet, I did not realize that much of my life would pass, and that still I could not release him who lies buried in the stone.

"For several years now the features of a man have been growing increasingly distinct in the surface of this marble, but I do not recognize him. At one time I thought perhaps it resembled the face of my learned father, he who went to his ancestors many years ago. But although the face is similar, it is also different. Moreover, my father, wise man that he was, never did himself know The Way. He frequently spoke of it, but said that few attain it."

Dao paused and waited to hear the Buddha speak to him, but all was silent within the shrine. He sat patiently, bowing at times toward the Buddha and raising his eyes at others, waiting some word of wisdom.

Finally, he sensed the tones of the Buddha's voice in his heart. They flashed a recollection of yesteryear. For the moment Dao felt as if he were young once again and just embarking on his lifelong quest. Perhaps now after he had labored so long, so diligently and so patiently, the Buddha would reward him with knowledge of The Way or of how it was to be acquired.

"My Son, you did well in struggling to bring back the white marble stone those many years ago. But lately you seem to have worked little in chipping away its outer coatings. Why have you not spent more time in this endeavor?"

A feeling of anguish and guilt came over Dao's heart. He realized that indeed he could have spent many hours, many days, many more moons in working at the stone. He did not know how to justify himself, but he felt that he must make the Buddha understand that he had truly striven with all his soul, that he had never forsaken his goal, and that he had remained faithful to his own best nature. Why was this not enough? Why was he now not rewarded? What more was demanded of him?

"Great Buddha, I could not work on the stone and be ever alone. That is why I took to wife the gracious lady who has been my constant companion, my joy and the mistress of my household. Man should not be required to live unto himself. He must share the trials and happiness which all things bring to each day. At times I would have returned to my work at the stone, but one of my little ones would come with the fever, and I would sit at night with him warding off evil spirits. At other times to get our food I must toil in the rice paddies, planting and harvesting. Then there were the fish to be caught in the nearby stream, the house to be repaired so as to please and keep happy my good wife. I searched in the ancient scrolls for wisdom as to The Way and, although I never found it there, I did acquire such knowledge that even a nephew of the emperor was sent to me for instruction.

"Often my wife and children would join me as we made journeys to the seaside to gather the shellfish and roast them over a fire. Many times I intended to chip more at the stone, but others sought my counsel, my time, my efforts. Only yesterday my little grandson climbed upon my knee and said, 'Grandfather, come play with

Adventures in Human Understanding

me.' Then he and I spent the rest of the day raking the fallen leaves in the garden, leaving the ground free for the coming snow.

"I wish so much to find The Way, but my entire life has been spent in doing all these things. I have even written good poetry, the scrolls of which are preserved in the library of the great university at Heiankyo. Perhaps I do not deserve to find The Way. I have neglected the work at the stone and am not worthy to achieve my quest. Tell me, oh Great One, is there something more I can still do while yet there is life in this body?"

Dao waited for the Buddha to say, "Foolish one, you have failed to do as I instructed you. You have wasted your life. You are not fit to find The Way. Go now and disturb me no more."

But such words did not come from the Buddha's mouth.

"My son, you have not done badly. But one more step is necessary. A fortnight from tomorrow the moon will rise over Mount Fuji at the stroke of midnight. Its light is often just right to see matters in the proper perspective, neither too bright nor too dim.

"Place the marble statue on the banks of the small island in your garden where it is clearly visible from the arching bridge. Let it look toward the sacred mountain. As the moon rises, gaze at the marble image. Concentrate on its features and, as you do, review your whole life. Bring to mind all your actions, worthy or despicable. Think of your ancestors, your parents, your childhood. Remember your struggles to bring the marble stone from the north and your efforts to earn your livelihood.

"Picture the face of your loving wife and each of your children. Bring back the memories of their victories and their heartaches. Recall the sickness which took some of them from you before they had achieved the fullness of their growth. Relive the journeys to the seashore and the feasts of the shellfish. Compute the pleasures and pains of your present existence, the aching in your bones, and the praises of the students whom you have instructed. Think of the great typhoon that leveled your home and the kind neighbors who helped you rebuild it. Think, My Son, think, and pass through your whole life once again. At the same time fix your gaze steadfastly upon the marble statue."

The voice of the Buddha faded to a whisper, so faint that Dao could no longer understand its words. Then there was silence. Quietly, he stretched his aching limbs and with a feeling of sadness began the long journey home. Disappointment filled his soul. The Buddha had told him to think and to change the location of the statue, but no word had he said about how to find The Way, nor what further he could do to recognize the image of the Knower-of-The-Way.

With weeping heart Dao returned to his house, but on passing its threshold he noticed the warm greeting of his wife somewhat cheered him. It almost removed his sadness—almost but not quite.

During the next fourteen days Dao laboriously moved the statue over to the island. This required that he build a raft of huge logs since the little bridge would not bear its immense weight. On the island's sandy shore he fashioned a pedestal of stones and seated the statue securely at its top, the face staring to the north-east where the mighty Fuji reared its snowy crest.

Once Dao had climbed to its peak. That was many years ago when he was young and agile. He remembered with a joyous lift the tremendous excitement he had experienced as he reached the summit and gazed out toward the mighty ocean which, as everyone knew, reached to the ends of the world. On the other side stretched the beauteous hills and valleys, the green slopes, terraced to enclose the small rice paddies. During the climb back down to the valley his spirit soared as it had never done before or since. There was something about Mount Fuji which was ennobling of the best in man. It was as if he who had attained its summit had received a blessing of the gods.

The evening of the full moon Dao seated himself on the arching bridge and waited. The quiet of the darkness scarcely concealed a rising tide of expectancy in his soul. Perhaps tonight he would achieve his quest. But the years had been so long, and he had been disappointed so often, that he stifled these hopes. Better that he wait and pray quietly, accepting whatever the gods had to offer, than that he expect success and fail.

A golden glow enveloped the lower reaches of the mountain. He could see where the thick forests stopped and the barren earth started. Then the whiteness of its peak became increasingly visible as the light behind it moved up and up. Dao held his breath. As his excitement mounted higher he almost fell into the pool. Suddenly a sliver of reddish gold appeared over the snow-capped cone. This gradually expanded until within a few minutes the entire yellowish orb was floating over the silvery peak like a toy balloon lifted by the wind.

Quickly he turned his gaze onto the features of the marble statue. There was the same long nose, the heavy eyebrows, the hair falling over the ears, the quizzical half-smile which so long he had studied.

The image in the statue seemed to be happy. He thought that whoever this represented looked both wise and strong. The Knower-of-The-Way displayed a serenity which said, "I am not afraid of my world. I can solve the problems it places on me. I can wait. I can wring from every moment of time that which is worthwhile in living and being. I like other people and respect them as I respect myself. I can give as well as receive. I can feel but am not a slave to my passions. The world is good. Life is good. I am good."

But then, why should not the Knower-of-The-Way be like this? Was this not what any person would feel and think if he had discovered The Way?

Dao felt empty. Why did the man in that statue have all these fine traits when he, Dao, had struggled all his life in ignorance of The Way? No word did the statue say to him. The harder he looked at the stone, the less it looked like anyone he had ever known.

Then he remembered the words of the Buddha. He was to review all the experiences of his own life while gazing at the features of the marble image. Gradually he sank into a reverie as the moon swam higher and higher in the ocean of the eastern sky.

Dao-Tsai and the White Marble Image

Bit by bit, piece by piece, almost as if they were being chipped from his being, tiny memories dropped into consciousness: The face of his beloved mother, she who was carried away by the white-clad mourners after coughing her last breath during the great pestilence. The kindly voice of his father who became both mother and father to him. The chidings when he was unworthy and the praise for accomplishments. The knowledge imparted to him by the elders and his own growing strength in games of skill. Through these he had learnt to accept equally the elation of victory and the barbs of defeat.

Much more came to his mind: His many years studying the poetry, the songs, the ancient scrolls left by his forefathers. The desire enkindled in him to find The Way and his great suffering in securing the white marble stone.

Then there passed before his eyes the face of his beloved wife, first as it looked tinted with the peach flower of youth, and later as the years added wisdom and a more majestic radiance to her features. He felt the tug at his heart as he realized the depth of her love. His children passed in review, their laughter and their tears.

The demon doll he had fashioned out of wood and horse hair and the amusement they all shared at its grotesque appearance. The cherry tree blooms of the springtime which filled his garden and the smell of his favorite incense. The golden rain of leaves flying from the spreading limbs of the maple trees in the forest and the clean, fresh whiteness of the winterscape after a storm. The successes of his children now occupying positions of respect and trust in various parts of the land and the tiny up-stretched hands of his grandchildren seeking to be carried on his shoulders down the garden path.

Then he recalled his own creations: The song which attracted the attention of the emperor, and the scroll of recognition which he had received at the court for its composition. Many hearts would be gladdened by it. Dao felt a sense of inner pride that it was his own brain-child.

His thoughts next passed to the present. The small cottage, shared now by only his wife and himself. It seemed to embody the utmost

Adventures in Human Understanding

of comfort and security from all that might be harmful. He pictured the small exchange of words, the warm tea prepared for his evening meal, and the slumber at eventide, often holding in his arms the gentle form of her who shared his heart.

All these images passed through Dao's mind while his entire being participated with feeling, with movement in their fullest understanding. He now felt so much closer to all that had happened to him in his life. But what had this to do with The Way to heaven? Here he was sitting on his bridge, and there was the statue across the pond on the sandy bank.

Once more he fixed his attention on the mass of white stone. There was nothing new in it, the same features, the same expression, and Dao felt a return of his sadness, his emptiness. The magic had not worked. He knew no more than before except perhaps a broadened view of his own nature, his past and his present. Tears tugged at the corners of his eyes. Was this all there was to be? Had the Buddha led him on a lifelong and futile search? Must he, too, join his ancestors ignorant of The Way?

Sadly he lowered his face and almost blankly stared into the dark blue waters below. The moon now neared the western sea, dancing and glimmering in the reflections from the pond. The white marble statue smiled at him like an enigmatic person whispering over and over again, "Who am I? Who am I? Who am I?"

In disgust Dao started to rise. Morning would soon arrive, and he wanted to return to his warm bed. However, just as he leaned over the pond another face appeared etched in white by the fading moonlight. He was so startled that at first he thought another must have been standing nearby, spying on him. Perhaps by his movement on the bridge, or perhaps because of the jumping of a frog, or maybe caused by a leaf floating down onto the water, a small school of golden carp were startled and began swimming from under the bridge out into the middle of the pool. As they swam, small waves were created. The moon, the white marble image and his own features rocked back and forth until at times they seemed to merge.

Dao-Tsai and the White Marble Image

With a start Dao sat up staring, unbelieving at what he perceived. The features of the marble statue and those of his own blended into a one-ness. The nose, the eyes, the mouth, the jaw, the hair, the neck. A dawning awareness overwhelmed his entire being. All of the pieces fit together like one massive puzzle. Like the bits he had carved from the white marble stone, the bits of memory from his life returned to a great unity. For the first time he comprehended the meaning of it all. He understood now the why of that which he had experienced, the relation with each other and with the fiber of his entire self, the purpose of the past, of the present and the direction of the future.

Dao knew whose image had been imprisoned in the stone. He fathomed with an overwhelming completeness himself and his own being. He understood who had always been the Knower-of-The-Way, and the words of the great Buddha that each man must find it for himself became fully clear to his senses.

An inner feeling of peace swept over him. Gone was the tension, the fears, the turmoil, the anxiety lest he fail, the guilt over his past, the doubts about his present and the gnawing feeling of unworthiness for his future.

Dao felt a kinship with the whole world, his ancestors, his past, his present, and all that would come in his future. It was as if his soul had merged with the essence of the universe itself. He was an integral part of the greater whole, the whole of all that existed.

It seemed to him that he was indeed the most fortunate man in the world. Whatever he needed to complete his life could be found here in his own home, with his loved ones, and in his own heart. He need not seek it elsewhere. Dao had found The Way—because he had always known The Way.

As the moon sank into the western sea, a burst of dawn swept away the darkness of night. The greens and golds of autumn never seemed so vivid. The sun was rising over Mount Fuji, and a new day was dawning. Quietly Dao rose and walked down the garden path to his house.

Thoughts of a Therapist: Analysis and Comment

Human nature has not changed much over the centuries. People in far away places and times have the same basic motivations we have today: Desires for health, prosperity, love, sex, achievements, security and the regard of one's associates.

For a complete life one needs a friend, an enemy, a love, a job and a home. One's "enemies" need not be people. They can be disease, injustice, poverty, pain or any of the problems with which we contend.

By what we are *for* (friends) and what we are *against* (enemies) we define the essence of what we *are*, our self. Judged by such standards, Dao-Tsai had achieved many of them by the time he reached old age.

Hearing about "The Way" as a youth from his father and others, he became highly motivated to accomplish that goal. "The Way" really means the achievement of one's major purposes, development of a stable self, satisfaction in one's existence, resolution of immaturities, unworthy aims, and the ability to face the future without fear (including one's own death).

Dao does not realize that "The Way" cannot be comprehended by future planning. It can be understood only *after* one has traversed it—in the past, not in the future. Nor does he realize that it must be discovered within one's own self, not in some outside object, person or deity.

The Buddha stresses the importance of commitment and perseverance. He gives Dao a task: to carve a statue of the "Knower-Of-The-Way" from a piece of marble. It will take most of his life.

While doing this, Dao leads a rewarding existence. He and his wife rear children who serve society, their community, the government, its military and their fellow countrymen.

He himself is a good citizen and promotes the values of his culture. He studies the historical lore of the past and becomes a successful, highly-respected teacher. In addition, he writes and publishes songs and poems. These are highly acclaimed and are retained in the great university. He takes personal satisfaction that they will "gladden many hearts."

Unbeknownst to him, he has been traversing "The Way" through all these years. It is therefore a shock, but a rewarding insight, when he discovers that it is he, himself, who has always unconsciously known "The Way."

The bits and pieces struck from the marble carving to reveal The-Knower-Of-The-Way are symbolic of the bits and pieces of his own existence; those which have developed his character.

Chapter 13

Quittin' Time

During an early scene in the movie *Gone With the Wind*, a group of slaves are working in the cotton field. It is evening, and one of the men shouts, "Quittin' Time." In great indignation the foreman proclaims, "I's de one dat sez, 'Quittin' Time. Quittin' Time!'"

In 1976, Gary Gilmore was convicted of the senseless murder of two young men. He was sentenced to death by the firing squad, the manner of executions in Utah at that time. Family, friends and lawyers appealed his conviction, seeking a lesser punishment. However, to the surprise of all, he opposed their efforts and demanded that he be executed.

Gilmore's execution posed a problem of indignation for society because he was saying "Quittin' Time" while his case was still on appeal. We didn't want him to be the one to say it, and his request for his own execution was embarrassing. Our revenge needs require a script in which the criminal is dragged screaming to the gallows, firing squad, electric chair or gas chamber.

In no way can we condone his vicious crimes, and our hearts go out to the victims and their families. But our real enemy should not be people. Rather it is the hatred and viciousness, which, like a pandemic disease, infects individuals and so pervades our society, that turns thousands of our young men (and women) each year into predatory animals. It is this disease, which inhabits human stuff, that we must find ways of eliminating, rather than the humans themselves. Man's cruelty to man resembles an infectious malady. It is passed from one person to another, from parent to child.

A simple way of viewing this problem is to divide the world into the good guys and the bad guys. As children, we were taught by the Western movies that good guys play fair and wear white hats. The villains fight dirty and wear black hats. We, the good guys, must eliminate them, the bad guys, and then everybody will live happily ever after.

From a broader perspective this entire Gilmore episode appears as a great tragedy for all concerned. Two young men of promise have been murdered. Grief and irreplaceable loss has been inflicted on their families. Violence has been stimulated. Society's hatreds have been exacerbated. And a man who was born an innocent baby, the same as all of us, has developed into a monster whose life is a menace to others.

One of the greatest human needs has been to see the good triumph over the bad, and we hope somehow we can put "the bad" into another person and then eliminate him. Unfortunately, such desires are in conflict with efforts to rehabilitate criminals.

Many of us do not want the felon rehabilitated. He serves us better if he becomes a vehicle into which we can pour all badness from society and from ourselves. It is purging to our own selves. We can then feel, "I am good; there goes the bad."

However, rehabilitation through death is also a tradition with us. Christ died to save the sins of others. Sydney Carton in *A Tale of Two Cities* relinquished his worthless life for the salvation of another. At funerals the dead person is always treated with respect.

Accordingly, many people validate their own existence through suicide when life is no longer valued because of excessive physical or mental pain, or because of the realization that the elimination of the badness within one's self can be accomplished only by a termination of one's entire being.

Society has tried ineffectively to change humans by punishment. Our prison system is a failure, either to deter or to rehabilitate. Penitentiaries do not make men penitent, nor do reformatories reform. The fact is that almost everyone perceives himself as the victim of forces over which he has no control, as a slave to society's pressures or to his own inner passions. Therefore, criminals consider themselves as having been "railroaded."

Rarely does a culprit say to the judge, "The verdict is fair; I am ready to accept the punishment." When this occurs, we do not perceive it as belated maturity, a development of social responsibility. We cannot tolerate letting a criminal garner to himself any of "the good." It must be that he is only staging a grandstand play; he is trying to be a hero, and we will not allow it.

Life should be valued for its quality measured in experiential time, not merely for its quantity measured in chronological time. When a person has come to recognize that his behavior is so loaded with badness that he is only a menace to his fellow men, and that his continued existence lacks any meaning, then let us permit him to dignify his exit and validate his membership in the human race. We can do this by accepting the one possession of value he has left to give, the removal from this world of a bad person who has brought only harm to others. Let us, like the Athenians of old, give him his desired cup of hemlock. For in so doing we once more affirm our belief in the dignity, the integrity of life and the possibility of redemption for all humans, good or bad.

The greatest and last possibility of growth toward maturity occurs to any individual who, recognizing that his existence no longer has value to himself or others, ceases to swim in futile desperation against the river of time. He rises out of his slavery and regains some measure of integrity when he can look up and announce to the world:

"It's Quittin' Time."

Chapter 14

The Clock

When Gilbert was a small boy, his father took him to the "Closing-Out" auction of a neighborhood furniture store. Dad never really intended to buy anything. The trip was part curiosity and part to show his son how auctions worked. Gilbert watched the spirited bidding with much interest. However, when this clock came up scarcely anybody seemed to want it. One bid, then silence.

"I got four dollars, gimme five, got four dollars, gimme five," shouted the red-faced auctioneer. "Who wants this fine grandfather clock for only five dollars?"

On an impulse Gilbert's father, thinking to get the betting started again, blurted out, "Five."

"Got five, gimme six, gimme six, gimme six. Going once. Going twice. Going three times—sold to Mr. Williams over there for five dollars."

"Well, I'll be damned," laughed his father. "What'll we do with it? We don't need another clock. Your mother will be upset."

When they got home he said, "Want to have it, Kid? We can hang it in your room." Delighted, Gilbert accepted.

So the half-grandfather clock was hung on the wall opposite Gilbert's bed. It was "half-grandfather" because the short pendulum was only 12 inches in length. It would swing back and forth like a real grandfather clock, but Gilbert found it must be wound often. So he wound it every morning when he first got out of bed.

None of his friends had a clock of their own. It made Gilbert feel important. He thought, "Clocks are very necessary. They tell you when to go to sleep, when to wake up, and when to leave for school. They measure when you are alive."

195

Adventures in Human Understanding

Over the years the clock had acquired another, very special message. Gilbert liked to hear its musical, bell-like ring. One day, while playing in the high school orchestra, he wondered just what was the pitch of its chime. So tuning the A string on his violin to his mother's piano, he checked its pitch the next time the clock struck.

"By golly! It's middle A." Something new. Excited, he accosted his father, "Look what I discovered, Dad!"

Dad, always the teacher, listened patiently to this burst of enthusiasm, then exclaimed, "That's how you do scientific research, Kid."

Gilbert never forgot. After that, unless he was sound asleep, whenever the clock started to chime, he counted with it, "A-one, A-two, A-three—."

Soon he made another observation. While curled up on the big easy chair just after lunch, he heard the clock's chime, and began dutifully counting, "A-one." It stopped ringing. That was all. One o'clock. It occurred to him that "A-one" also meant the best.

Dad always said. "Do your best, achieve, discover new things, help other people, and be A-one."

So whenever the clock would start chiming, Gilbert imagined it was Dad saying to him, "Do your best. Be A-one."

In high school he took courses from his father. If he didn't make the honor roll it was because his Dad was the one who had given him the B grade. That occurred two times.

Now, many years later, Gilbert always thought "A-one" when the clock started chiming. But he couldn't believe that he, himself, was really A-one. He decided at least he deserved a B-plus.

Whenever the clock struck, he could almost hear his Dad's gentle, teaching voice: "The measure of a man is how much he can be trusted, and whether he gives back to the world. There's too many takers these days."

The Clock

[handwritten: "to be trusted" / "mum?"]

This afternoon he started his nap early. When he was awakened by the clock's chimes he began counting as usual. "A-one, A-two, A-three, A-four. Four o'clock. How come I slept so long? Must have been very tired. Suzie comes home any time now. She promised she would have a surprise."

There was a crunch outside as the big yellow school bus ground to a stop on the ice-covered street in front of the house. A few seconds later the porch door burst open.

"Grandpa! Grandpa! Look what I made today. Miss Stewart said it was the best one she had ever seen."

Suzie fished in her bag and pulled out a tea-mat woven with brown and red straws. Just the thing for the dining-room table. Mother would be pleased. Gilbert answered enthusiastically, "It's beautiful. I'll bet it took you a long time."

Blonde-haired Suzie was always excited when she went to kindergarten, and equally so when she returned in the afternoon. Life was one great big, frothy bubble of interesting things to learn and do.

Gilbert felt younger when Suzie was around—reminded him of his own boyhood and the pleasure he felt in telling his father about his achievements of the day. Dad never failed to reward him with approval, at least when the accomplishment had value.

"Grandpa, can we read some more tonight?"

Suzie always knew the answer would be "yes," but she asked anyway. She could almost read alone, even though she was only four years old.

Just before bedtime she and Grandpa "read" together. Putting on her red pajamas Suzie climbed into the big, plush chair under the clock in his room. It was large enough (just barely) to accommodate a little girl and a skinny old man.

Often it was from the big red book labeled "Nursery Tales." Sometimes they read together; sometimes Suzie by herself. The rest of the time she followed the lines while Grandpa read. Then

Suzie would just stare at the type. When curious, she would, pointing, ask, "What does that word there mean?" After that, she could generally recognize it again the next time it occurred.

They finished reading the story of "Cinderella." The clock began to chime. Suzie knew what that meant. Reluctantly she cooperated. "One, two, three, four, five, six, seven, eight—nine." Nine o'clock and time for bed. Now came the last game. She stuck her foot out. Pausing a moment, Gilbert said, "This little pig went to market," pinching the big toe. Then, "This little pig stayed home," as he pulled on the second toe. Suzie waited breathlessly, knowing well what was supposed to come next. "This little pig had roast beef," the middle toe, followed by, "This little pig had none."

Gilbert paused a few seconds before the last one, and Suzie, with wide-eyed expectation, crouched like their cat, Samantha, ready to pounce on Caesar, the squirrel in the back yard.

Then, pinching her little toe, he shouted, "This little pig cried, 'Wee, Wee, Wee,' all the way home."

Midst squeals of glee and roaring laughter, he announced, "Now to bed, you rascal." She danced downstairs.

"Mama, Mama, I'm ready to be tucked in." Scurrying to her room, Suzie scrambled into bed. Marilyn followed, pulled up the covers, kissed her, and inquired, "What did you and Grandpa read tonight?"

"About Cinderella. I like a story best if it ends with everything just the way it's supposed to be."

Mother nodded. "Good night, Dear." Then, turning off the light, she closed the door. In five minutes all was quiet.

Gilbert was left with his thoughts. "Suzie will make a great teacher. I'm glad these young people are coming along. They'll take over when we're gone."

He lay down. Propping his head up in bed with a pillow, he picked up a dog-eared copy of Keegan's *The First World War*, and resumed reading "The Battle of the Somme."

He recalled his own military experience in World War II and often thought, "Stand straight. Shoulders back. 'Ten—shun." He was not going to be one of those old codgers who were bent over. It hurt his arthritis to straighten up, but it made him feel more like a man.

The Somme battle having been finished (with no victory for either the British or the Germans), Gilbert let the book slip out of his hands as he dozed off without changing to his pajamas.

He awoke with a start. What time was it? Today he hadn't been feeling well. Probably just another case of the indigestion he often experienced when he had eaten too much or snacked on too much chocolate. At dinner, he had gobbled an extra helping of plum pudding.

"Oh well, an Alka Seltzer would fix it." It also worked this time too—almost. However, even two additional aspirin tablets didn't quite stop that pain in his chest.

Six months ago he and Martin, seven years older than Suzie, had been playing basketball, throwing the ball at the hoop he had rigged up above the garage door. The action was spirited and, after he had failed to make a long shot, Gilbert felt excruciating pain and difficulty breathing. Martin called his mother. Marilyn took him immediately to the Community Hospital.

Dr. Muggeridge sternly lectured him, "Listen, Old Fellow, you can't be playing such strenuous games. You've had a mild heart attack. I'm going to keep you in the hospital for a couple of days—just to observe."

Gilbert grumped, "I don't want to go to a damned hospital. That's where people die."

Dr. Muggeridge patiently continued, "You've been around a long time. That ticker has taken a lot of wear and tear. No more basket-

Adventures in Human Understanding

ball for you. A walk every day—and cut down on rich, fatty foods. Take it easy, and you can last for years."

Of course, both Marilyn and Eleanor, when she was alive, had also harped at him about his exercise and diet. However, Dr. Muggeridge was one person whose scoldings you took seriously. When he said something it meant business. Gilbert had "behaved himself" and cut down on the chocolate.

It had been five years since Gilbert's wife, Eleanor, had slipped on the icy steps. Fractured her femur. The operation went well, but two months later she fell again. The pin broke out. After that, she never recovered. Just drifted away.

He had married her, a petite little redhead, right out of high school, and they had been in love almost 60 years. He adored her. Every morning when she first opened her eyes he would reach over, pat her and say, "Good morning, Beautiful," and at night it was, "Good night, Pretty Girl." She would purr, like Samantha.

Once they saved almost enough money for a cruise to the Bahamas. But his hospitalization and surgery for gall bladder had taken most of it. They settled for a trip to Disneyland.

When she died Gilbert was devastated. He retreated to the bedroom and cried all day for several months. Agnes Worthington, who lost her husband two years before, invited him for Sunday dinner. Although she was reputed to be the best cook in town, he turned her down.

People meant well. They thought he ought to "snap out of it." But something in him insisted that he had to go over and over the good times he and Eleanor had enjoyed together. "Mourning" was healing, but he didn't realize it then. In time, he felt "cried-out."

Ultimately, the children, all seven of them, decided he shouldn't live alone. They "persuaded" him to sell the old family home and move into the spare room in Bill and Marilyn's place. Gilbert protested. "I can take care of myself." The family prevailed.

When the old house was sold he kept only his bed, the big easy chair, and the clock, then settled into a lonely existence—which continued until Suzie arrived.

He was wide awake now. A million thoughts went rushing through his head: His life with Eleanor, their children, his teaching years, when he was a little boy—and his father.

One summer day, when school was out, he and "Huffy," his best friend, had gone skinny dipping in the river and were taking it easy on the grassy bank. They both were thirteen. Huffy asked, "What do you want to be when you're grown?" Gilbert replied, "All I want is to be famous, maybe President, make a million dollars, and marry the prettiest girl in the world."

"Ha!," replied Huffy skeptically. "You don't want much."

Now Gilbert lay quietly musing to himself. How much of those immature, childish dreams had he accomplished?

Teachers made little money. He hadn't become President, and even though he considered Eleanor very pretty, she hadn't been the beauty queen in high school.

"I guess I didn't make it. I'm not A-one."

His thoughts turned toward those days of teaching. He had graduated with a bachelor's degree. Jobs were scarce, so when he received a letter from Arlie Perkins, Superintendent of Hillsdale Schools, offering a job teaching mathematics, science and music, he eagerly accepted.

No contract came. Perplexed, he went to see Mr. Perkins, who was very evasive. "I think you better talk with Mrs. Ripton, chairman of the school board. She is the cook at Andy's Grill."

Mrs. Ripton, a stern-faced 60-year-old, looked at him disapprovingly over the horn-rimmed glasses, which were pulled down over her nose.

Adventures in Human Understanding

"Mr. Williams. We understand you have played in a dance orchestra. We have a God-fearing community here, and we don't want our young people taught bad morals."

Gilbert was stunned. It never occurred to him that earning part of his college expenses playing for dances would cause any trouble getting a teaching job. He replied respectfully, "Well, Mrs. Ripton, I don't smoke or drink. And I played for dances only to help with college expenses. I won't be playing any dances when I teach in Hillsdale." Mrs. Ripton just stared over her glasses and said, "Hm."

Mr. Perkins told him to get character references. So he asked Professor Preston, with whom he had studied at the nearby college. Professor Preston and Dr. Boone, the college's president, drove in Boone's old Ford the 18 miles to Hillsdale. They talked with Mrs. Ripton. He received his contract.

Next, he remembered the time when Harley Baker had opened Gilbert's classroom door just after school was dismissed for the day. Harley was almost in tears because he thought he'd have to drop out of school.

"Harley, I don't see why you can't turn in homework assignments like the rest of the class."

"It's this way, Mr. Williams. I live six miles from town. The bus doesn't come our direction. I have to get up early to help milk ten cows. Then I walk to school. After school, I walk home and help with the ten cows. Dad needs me. I'm sorta tired then, and I just feel like going to bed."

Gilbert resisted the impulse to say, "You pass." He knew he must not grant favors. He had to think of all his students. "Harley, could you come in after you finish lunch? I'll help you get a passing grade." Harley smiled. At the end of the year there was a C grade in Algebra on his report card.

Then there was Russell, who ran out of a counseling session and headed down the street. Gilbert had chased him almost a half mile

The Clock

before he slowed up and could be convinced to stay in school. Gilbert thought, "I wonder if teachers have to do that these days?"

Many similar incidents came to mind. And when each one did, he had a distinct feeling of pride and pleasure. In fact, one year he'd been named "Teacher-of-the-Year" for the whole county. Maybe he really was better than just a B-plus teacher.

At 69 (and many hundred students later), Gilbert decided it was time to retire. His arthritis hurt, and he was so sleepy at night he didn't want to grade any more papers. He turned in his resignation.

The Superintendent, Arlie Perkins, called him into the office. "What's this business about retiring, Gib? I know you're over age, but we can't get new, young teachers today. Those who are competent won't accept the salaries we can offer. How about staying one more year?"

Gilbert wanted to say, "No," but he couldn't. He just couldn't. So he was 70 when finally he'd cleaned out his desk.

One day a few years ago, the phone had rung. Answering it, Gilbert heard a familiar voice ask "Is this Mr. Williams, who taught in Hillsdale high school?

"Yes."

"Well, this is Lloyd Condon. I'm the guy you helped buy a cornet for the band. You also arranged a paper route for me."

Gilbert beamed all over. "Lloyd? Of course I remember you. I'm delighted you called. How did you locate me?"

"It wasn't easy. I finally found you in the State Directory," Lloyd replied.

Gilbert was very pleased that one of his students had gone to all this trouble.

Adventures in Human Understanding

"Dad didn't think I needed any more schooling. He wanted me to work on the ranch. If it hadn't been for that paper route, I'd have dropped out of school."

Gilbert recalled that Lloyd was very bright but mischievous. There were some folks in town who predicted he'd get in trouble. Gilbert had tweaked the boy's interest in science and also taught him the cornet, which he played in the school band. After that his whole attitude had changed.

Lloyd continued. "Did you know after I graduated I went to college—got a bachelor's degree? During World War II, I became a Major and was Administrative Officer for a large Army Hospital in Italy. Then I was a high school principal in California until I retired."

You could have knocked Gilbert over with a feather. He struggled to find something to say. "During the War I was only a Sergeant, Lloyd. If we'd met I would have had to salute you." His feeling of pride became very intense.

Lloyd continued. "Next month our class is holding a 50-year reunion. They wanted me to see if you could come and give a talk." Gilbert was speechless. This was about the nicest thing that had ever happened to him. He finally mumbled an acceptance.

It was Saturday in mid July. The class held its 50-year reunion in conjunction with the county fair. A big parade was scheduled. The high school band (once his band) would march. The parade would include a line of antique automobiles. He could have his pick of one in which to ride. He chose a red, 1929 Buick Convertible, the kind he had admired as a boy, but which his family couldn't possibly afford. The parade went down Hillsdale's Main Street. Gilbert didn't recognize anybody, but he waved anyway. Many hands waved back.

That evening he and twenty-five of his old students met for a picnic dinner. It started to rain, so they moved all the food into the high school gym. A flood of memories overwhelmed him. There was the stage on which his orchestra and chorus had performed the operetta, *The Gypsy Rover*, which he had directed. Just before dinner many of them told stories he had forgotten—some of which he didn't recall even happening.

"Do you remember," remarked one bewhiskered old fellow, "when we graduated, I didn't have a suit to wear? I was ashamed to go. You loaned me your dark blue one. I'll never forget that."

Gilbert wasn't sure, although he did recall he had owned two suits, a brown one for everyday class and a blue one for teaching Sunday School.

Another of his old students approached and shook his hand. "You remember me—and the water witching? I'm Louie. You sure gave me a rough time, I never did convince Dad."

Gilbert remembered. All the wells in the county had been located by "water witching." Holding a forked peach branch in front, you walked until it turned down. That's where you dug and found your well. Gilbert had asked the county surveyor about it, who informed him, "Of course they found water. There's a natural table underneath all the farms. You can't miss." Gilbert had not told the class of this, but instead had suggested "a scientific experiment" to settle the matter. Louie mentioned in class that his father witched most of the wells in the community, and that he had also taught Louie how to do it. He, Louie, would be glad to demonstrate.

The next day Louie brought his peach branch to school. The class traipsed out into the school yard, which was surrounded by fields.

"Now Louie, show us how you do water witching." Louie held the forked peach branch in front of him and proclaimed, "It goes like this." He started walking across the field behind the school. Gilbert and the class followed. After a while, the branch turned down. Louie pointed. "That's where you get water if you dig." Gilbert put a peg in the ground.

Louie backed off from the peg and approached it from several different directions. In each case the branch turned down when he got close. There was a general nodding of acceptance. Louie had proved his point.

Adventures in Human Understanding

Gilbert raised another question. "Now Louie, you're sure the branch is being pulled down by the water, and you don't have anything to do with it?"

Louie felt very confident. "That's right. It's the water."

"Well, if that's the case you won't object to doing it again—blindfolded?"

Louie was surprised, as well as all the other students. He'd never been asked this before. After a slight hesitation he replied, "Of course."

The group then wandered around the field, Gilbert leading the procession and holding the arm of the blindfolded Louie.

To the surprise of Louie and the rest of the class, the peach branch never turned down twice in the same place. When confronted with this he threw it away in utter disgust, declaring, "I'd never convince Dad of this."

At the next quiz Gilbert posed the question, "Do you believe in water-witching?" There were nineteen "No"s and one "Yes," with the added note, "Louie just ain't a good witch."

After this session Gilbert wondered, "Did I hurt Louie? He certainly was embarrassed in front of his classmates. Maybe he would have an argument with his Dad, or his father would get angry?" Nothing bad occurred, and Louie was just as friendly.

Others of his old students wanted to talk with him. One of the "girls" approached. She was gray-haired, bespectacled and grandmotherly now. That face looked familiar.

"Can I have a moment with you, Mr. Williams?" They all addressed him as "Mr. Williams," even though he called them by their first names. "Do you remember me, Mary Ellen Ripton? That day when you taught about evolution in the science class we almost walked out. I told Reverend McAlister, our minister, what you said. He explained that to get the truth, I only had to read the first book in the Bible. If you told us we came from monkeys, then you were an atheist, and we didn't have to listen to you. We were not going to come to your class any more if you hadn't changed matters the next day."

Gilbert recalled that almost-crisis, but he hadn't known how bad it was. As the science teacher, he knew he had to teach about evolution in biology class. He wondered whether Mrs. Ripton would get him fired afterward. He had thought a long time and finally decided he'd try a compromise Friday, which the class might accept.

So he had told them, "Evolution never said God did not create the earth, but maybe evolution was just His way of doing it. You remember in the book of Genesis it says that the earth was first covered with water. Then the herb yielding seed, and the tree yielding fruit developed. The dry land next appeared, and the animals came. First fish in the oceans, then winged animals, then all the other beasts. Finally, it says that man was the last one created. Isn't that what the Bible says?"

There was a general nodding of agreement. Kids in that community knew their Bibles.

"Well, that's almost the same order in which evolution says it happened."

Mary Ellen had raised her hand. She was not about to let him off the hook easy. "But in the Scriptures it says He did all this in seven days. Does evolution claim the Holy Bible is wrong?" Gilbert knew this question was coming. He had already framed his answer.

"No. But did you ever think that we measure a day by one revolution of the earth? At the beginning of creation there wasn't any earth to revolve. So perhaps God's day is much longer than ours. Couldn't God in his magnificence have had a day that was as long as a million years of our days, or even a billion years? That would be in line with what scientists have found." Then to make it more convincing, he added, "Including the dinosaurs, whose pictures are in your biology book?"

Adventures in Human Understanding

Well, it wasn't exactly the truth, but it wasn't a complete lie either. Mary Ellen's face had changed from a challenging frown, to one of puzzlement, thoughtfulness, and finally almost an acceptance. Gilbert knew the worst was behind. Everybody came to school Monday. He didn't get a letter from Mr. Perkins saying Mrs. Ripton wanted him fired.

So it went throughout the reunion day. There was a standing ovation after his post-dinner speech. Gilbert felt very appreciated, very respected.

A cloud remained. Somebody mentioned that Wilbur Groves, one of the class members, had joined the Air Force during the War, and had been shot down over Germany.

Once, in algebra class, Gilbert noticed during an exam that Wilbur, a very poor student who sat in the back row, was copying from Hester, who sat next to him. The more he watched Wilbur, the more upset Gilbert became. This had to stop. It was unfair. No good teacher would knowingly permit cheating.

He strode down the aisle. Stopping in front of Wilbur's desk, he grabbed the boy's paper and tore it up, announcing in a loud voice, "We don't tolerate cheating in this class." Gilbert felt a great sense of righteousness—like Moses smashing the tablets. Wilbur cowered back into the woodwork of his chair. A hush enveloped the room. Several looked at Wilbur. Nobody looked at Gilbert.

The next day Wilbur didn't come to school. In fact, he never came to school anymore. Gilbert felt terrible. By humiliating a student in front of his classmates he had destroyed the boy's chance for an education. He would never do that again. Throughout the rest of his life, whenever he thought of Wilbur, Gilbert felt bad.

The clock's chime returned Gilbert to reality. He was not alert enough to start the counting. Some moonlight filtered through the window blind. He could see the clock. "twelve o'clock, midnight. Almost a new day."

He sank back into his reveries. That remark to Huffy about being famous? He wasn't President. But he was very important to a lot

The Clock

of people. Those "kids" and many more had passed through his classes for 40 years. Maybe that was all the fame he needed. What difference did it make whether it was a whole nation or only a few hundred kids? They respected him; they touted him, they loved him—and there were many more Lloyds than Wilburs. What more fame did he need?

A feeling of contentment poured over his entire body, drenching him like a cool swim on a summer day. Almost all of his concerns now made sense. Almost all.

"But what about the million dollars? Why hadn't he acquired wealth? What was money for?" he asked himself.

Another part of him replied, "To buy pleasures and happiness? Old man Quigley owned the biggest house in town. Folks said he made a million in the stock market. But his wife had left him because he was abusive, and his kid was in jail. He sure wasn't getting any pleasure out of his money."

Gilbert compulsively chewed his thoughts like a dog with a bone. "Why do we need money to be happy? Why do people measure wealth by how much money you made?"

More and more the realization swept over Gilbert that he had all he ever needed, all he really wanted. This train of thought led to an exciting realization: Even though he wouldn't be leaving much to his children, he was truly a very wealthy man. This revelation electrified his entire being.

"Wow! I'm rich! All these years I've been acquiring wealth and didn't know it. Well, I'll be damned." He relaxed back into the pillow.

In a half-dream, half-awake condition Gilbert felt as if he were now in his father's classroom. It was the last day of school. He was alone. All his classmates had left. Dad was returning the final examination papers. Sluggishly, as if in slow motion, he trudged toward his father's desk. Dad just sat up there, so immense, so majestic, almost like Zeus on Olympus.

Adventures in Human Understanding

Gilbert thought. This would be it. His father would tell him now just where he stood. The final grade. He would know whether he was on the honor roll—or not.

It seemed ages before father reached over and handed down his paper. Gilbert tried to open it and see what grade he had made.

"Bong," the clock chimed. Startled, Gilbert opened his eyes halfway. Its sound seemed to be as weary as he was. The single musical tone reverberated and kept repeating itself as if it had floated from thousands of miles away. Its voice was firm, but gentle and tender. "A-one. A-one. A-one."

Gilbert looked up at the clock. Yes, there was his father's face, the strong but kindly smile which had always guided him. Dad seemed pleased and was nodding. So calm. So peaceful. Gilbert took a deep breath and settled back on the pillow. He understood. Yes, now he understood.

It occurred to him there was one more thing he needed to do. One more thing—that last teenage boast, then everything would be complete.

He already knew the answer, but just to be sure he tried to roll over on his right side. The body didn't budge. His arms had no feeling, and he couldn't move them. Never mind. The pain was gone. In its place was a rosy glow. Even though he couldn't stir, he felt as if every fiber of his self was suffused with joy—sheer joy. He was young again, vigorous, powerful, and he could do anything he wanted.

In his "mind's eye" he turned to the right, reached over and patted the other pillow while whispering softly, very softly, "Good Night, Pretty Girl." Then he smiled.

Marilyn was stirring a bowl of batter when she heard Suzie shout from the top of the stairs.

"Mama! I want to wear my new dress today. O.K.?" Marilyn had hoped to save it for some special occasion, but she tried to let Suzie make as many decisions as possible. It developed independence in children.

"O.K., dear. If that's what you want."

A few minutes later Suzie came sliding down the banister.

"Miss Stewart told us how pollywogs lose their tails, grow legs, and turn into frogs. She promised to bring a bowl of them today, so we could see it happen."

Marilyn was amused. "What little it took to please children."

Bill was absorbed in the Morning Bulletin, covering the latest breakdown of peace negotiations between the Israelis and the Palestinians, when he heard Marilyn say, "Suzie, go call Grandpa. Tell him we're having his favorite pancakes today." Suzie took the stairs two steps at a time.

A minute later she rushed downstairs. "Mama! Daddy! Grandpa's asleep, and he won't wake up! I knocked on the door. He didn't answer, so I went in. He's on the bed with all his clothes on."

A look of alarm crossed Marilyn's face. "Bill." she yelled, "Come quick! Something's wrong with Dad."

They both dashed up the stairs. One glance and they knew immediately what had happened. The whole family clustered around. Everybody but Suzie was crying.

"What's the matter with Grandpa?" she anxiously inquired.

Marilyn turned away to hide her tears. "He was very old, Susie, and he's just gone to sleep." Suzie felt she shouldn't ask any more questions right now.

As they filed out Bill said to Marilyn, "Do you know what time it happened?

"No. I slept soundly all night."

Adventures in Human Understanding

"I noticed his old clock had stopped at one o'clock," Bill observed. "Probably forgot to wind it yesterday."

Marilyn thought, "Forgot? That's strange. He's never forgotten to wind it before."

At breakfast nobody spoke, not even Martin who was usually very talkative. Suzie sensed that maybe she was not supposed to speak—like in church. Everyone seemed to be engrossed in their own thoughts. When they left the table, there were two pancakes still on the tray.

Martin had already left for school and, as Bill was putting on his coat, Marilyn remarked, "I'll make the arrangements, after I clean up."

Suzie wondered what her mother meant by "arrangements."

The tears kept coming, and Marilyn felt the need to be by herself. "Hurry up, dear. Get your coat. Here's your lunch pail."

Suzie knew something was wrong. But it was five minutes before the bus was due, and she had some questions on her mind.

"Mama, when's Grandpa going to wake up?"

"He's not going to wake up, dear. He's going to stay asleep."

Suzie seemed puzzled. "Won't he wake up and read some more stories with me?"

"No, dear. He's lived a long time, and he was very tired. You know how you feel when you get too tired and sleepy." Suzie looked concerned, so Marilyn added, "He's done so many things. I guess he just didn't want to stay awake any longer. Perhaps he felt worn out."

"Well, why was he smiling when we saw him?"

That stumped Marilyn a moment. She replied, "I think that's because he is happy."

Suzie sat quietly for awhile. Then she brightened up. "Well, if he went to sleep because he was too tired, and he wants to stay there, and if he's happy, then everything's just the way it's supposed to be—isn't it, Mama?"

Marilyn thought, "How wise we are when we are only four." She replied, "I think you're right, Dear."

There were two honks outside. The big yellow bus pulled up. Suzie yelled, "I'm coming. I'm coming," and rushed out the door. She was breathless when she reached the bus. Looking back, while standing on the steps, she waved briskly to her mother.

So life goes. Marilyn rewound the clock and made the "arrangements." Bill worked at the office. Suzie showed off her new, pink dress at school, and Miss Stewart told her how nice she looked. Martin was elected Captain of the school basketball team. The pollywogs all grew into frogs. Suzie became a teacher—and everything turned out just the way it's supposed to be.

Thoughts of a Therapist: Analysis and Comment

The most important issue here is the powerful impact a parent's relationship with a child can have on the young person's career and life. Gilbert's father provided a role model, spending time and guiding him. He was a "pal" as well as a father.

Had the father been a criminal, an immature individual, or one holding destructive values, the effect could have been just as profound, but Gilbert would have turned out much differently.

Parents do not appreciate the power they have for influencing a young child, not by rules, rigid discipline and punishment, but by attention, care, and time spent together. Some parents, unfortunately, discover this family resource only after it is too late.

Adventures in Human Understanding

Gilbert never forgot this modeling by his father, nor his tradition of community service (teaching), which he, Gilbert, transmitted to his little granddaughter, Suzie.

Note the contrast here of parent behavior with that of Gus, Goodwin's father in the story of "The Nerd," or Roger, the father of Quentin in the tale of "The Cuckoo Bird's Egg."

Second only to parents and immediate family is the impact of teachers on the lives of our children. In the early grades, where young people are most malleable, the power of the teacher as a model of maturity, adjustment and wise behavior is at a peak. In this society, where both parents often work outside the home, teachers may actually be in contact with the children longer hours than their parents.

If the teacher is patient, kindly, nurturant and understanding, her young charges thrive, and are more likely to become responsible, producing citizens.

On the other hand, teachers like Miss McFarland, in the story of "The Nerd," by her unthinking correction of a simple misspelling error, inflicted a lifelong hurt on Goodwin. Similar was the effect on Wilbur by Gilbert's handling of cheating. Accuracy of learning and honesty in taking tests can be taught without devastating child egos.

In high school and college, instructors have great influence over a pupil's choice of occupation. Almost everyone can remember an interesting (sometimes brilliant) teacher who inspired them, often into their present careers.

More time should be spent evaluating the maturity, integrity and social responsibility of teachers—not only their mastery of subject matter. Even Mrs. Ripton was aware of teacher influence on character.

Another issue here is the ability to reconcile unrealistic goals of youth with accomplishments as an adult. Before dying, Gilbert accepts that as an imperfect human he has not achieved all his aims. However, he reviews his life and decides he has done a fairly good job—in spite of an occasional bad move, such as his treatment of Wilbur. He redefines those early goals more realistically and can accept that he deserves the "A-one" grade signaled by his father's clock.

Finally, this story emphasizes the inevitability of life's stages: Childhood, adolescence, maturity, old age, the passing of "the mantle" to future generations, and the desirability of making peace with one's self before leaving. Of such is happiness built. Then, as 4-year-old Suzie put it, "everything's just the way it's supposed to be."

Part IV

The Promise of Life

Chapter 15

The Golden Journey[1]

Jack D. Watkins[2]

Many years ago, three men set out on a journey to seek wisdom. One of them was blind and could not see the way. Another was deaf, could see, but could not hear directions. Still another, the third, could see and hear but was mute and could not speak to transmit directions.

The three would make the journey together. But how? Each one was incapable of making it by himself. After many false starts and much obvious frustration, the three sat down by the roadside to reflect upon their dilemma. The blind man was frustrated because his acute sense of hearing always grasped directions from each passerby, but the other two could not comprehend his verbal communications. The second man had an acute sense of sight, but was terribly frustrated in not being able to hear or accurately convey the directions to the other two. The third man was perhaps the most frustrated in that he could see the way, and hear the directions, but alas could not communicate with the other two. The three seekers of wisdom sat together in solemnity. They bowed their heads in deep contemplation, waiting for an answer.

Suddenly, after a long silence, a Voice came from the skies. It was a Voice that reverberated through thunder and lightning and could be seen by the blind man. It was also a Voice that somehow could even be heard by the deaf man. And finally, it was a Voice that could be understood and acknowledged verbally by the mute man.

---

[1] This story was first read on Dec. 25th, 1986 in Portland, Oregon as a Christmas sermon by the Reverend Alan Deale, Pastor of the First Unitarian Church.
[2] Jack D. Watkins is the son of John G. Watkins and an independent author in his own right.

"Listen to me now! Oh, Three-on-a-Journey. You have failed to make any progress because one important ingredient is missing among you. Now, form a circle and join your hands. Squeeze your hands tightly and feel the result. The answer that lies in each of your hearts is the same. It is called "trust." For without trust between each of you, this journey cannot be made. With it you can succeed, if you are also able to learn three rules of gold on the way. The journey will be hard and long, but a great richness awaits you at the end. Now! Be on your way. And with the new-found trust that you have discovered, rely on each other's talents. For, whether through sound, sight or touch, it will be your blessing that one sees no evil, one hears no evil, and the third speaks no evil.

The journeymen joined hands in a circle as the Voice continued. "I give you, as a gift for your learning of trust, one camel to accompany you on the journey. You must all decide how he may best assist you along the way. He is spindly of leg, humped of back, and short of temper. But he has a staying power and a long endurance for the journey. Now! Be off on your way." With this, the Voice abruptly stopped.

Suddenly, the camel appeared at the journeymen's campsite. They immediately made fast their preparations to undertake the trip. The men fashioned saddlebags from their camp equipment and clothing. With these lashed firmly on the beast's humps, they loaded on all the goods from their camp, until there was a small mountain of things piled on the camel, leaving one decision that would have to be made. Which one of the three men would lead the way and for how long? After much disagreement, the three men decided to apply what they had learnt from the Voice. A circle once again was formed and the three joined hands, squeezing tightly. A further measure of trust seemed to emerge. They all smiled.

Since only one of the three at a time could ride on the camel, the other two would walk on either side of the beast, holding the bridle as security and to guide the creature. In this way, no one would have to lead; and, furthermore, each of the three could take a rest periodically by riding atop the hump. It seemed like a splendid idea, and so the journeymen and the camel began their expedition.

The Golden Journey

Suddenly, after many long days into the trip, a violent sandstorm burst forth and seized the travelers. In its rage the storm lashed them furiously until they were sore and weary from its impact.

Afterwards, when the storm had subsided and a calm existed, the men found themselves in a total state of confusion. They all sat down to wait for what they felt was sure death, for in the storm's fury their only full water jug was lost.

The end for them all seemed near. Then, unexpectedly, the Voice came, with its thunder and lightning. The pilgrims immediately stood up to receive its message.

"Journeymen Three! See and hear me, bright and clear. You have failed to learn the first of the rules of gold, of which I spoke. Just now, you were ready to die, because you felt nature had defeated you. You lacked an important ingredient in the fabric of mankind, something that guides you in life, wherever you may go. It is called "Faith." It can be faith in your fellowmen, whether travelers in your party, or not. It can also be faith in yourselves to succeed. But, perhaps, it can also be faith in something greater than even your fellowmen, or yourselves. Let us say that it can be faith of one, or more, of all these things. Now, before I leave, let me say I cannot find faith for you, but you can find it for yourselves. If you have anything, and it seems little at this point, you will now do what you will."

The three men beheld these enlightening words in awe. They joined hands once again in the circle of trust. The desert breeze that wafted up now found three heads bowed and six trembling hands joined.

After a while, through the talents of each (vision, hearing and touch), they could discern over the next hill a wondrous place. Tall palm trees ringed an azure pool of water below them. The men filled their remaining empty water jugs and smiled at the lesson of faith they had learnt.

Once refreshed, they resumed their journey, one mounted atop the camel and the other two on each side, grasping the bridle firmly with only the camel seeming to lead.

Adventures in Human Understanding

The longest and most arduous stretch of the pilgrimage was now to be undertaken. The blistering sun of the afternoon and the frigid cold of night exhausted both the wayfarers' minds and bodies. Day after day, the rotation of the three atop the camel took place.

After several days it became apparent that they had lost their way in the vast sands of the desert. The three sat down in despair and once again prepared for the end. They all agreed that it seemed pointless to go on.

Then, at the moment of their deepest despair, the Voice made known its presence once more to them. In a booming voice like thunder from the heavens it proclaimed: "Listen, you travelers! You still have not learned the second of the rules of gold. You sit there huddling in self-pity and defeatism. You fail to consider one of man's most important needs. It is called "Hope." No matter how black the night may seem, or how lost you may feel, if you can have hope you need never despair. I cannot give you that quality of hope, but it can be felt and nourished by each of you. I leave you now. Do what you will. Remember one last thing! If you do find Hope, it is not the last of the rules of gold. I cannot tell you anything about the final rule. You will all have to find it, each in your own way. I speak no more."

With faith now resurging, the firm hand-grips in their circle of three bespoke a new resolution. They bowed their heads together for a moment, then lifted them upward as if in a great cry of hope.

Suddenly, in the pale blue of dusk painted over the desert sands, three heads bobbed in excitement as they saw a bright shimmering star. It was as if a beacon had been sent to guide them. They knew now that they had found Hope and that their hope had been rewarded. They also decided that, to save their energies from the blistering heat, they would travel by night.

The blind, deaf and mute voyagers now set out in the moonlight, convinced they had all the knowledge needed to reach the end of their travels. All they would have to do would be to trust themselves, have Faith and Hope and follow that beautiful beckoning star in the heavens above.

The Golden Journey

But, totally unexpected by them, there was a huge chain of mountains blocking the way, jagged peaks thrust into the heavens above. However, they did become aware of one narrow canyon which might lead to their final destination. As the three men came nearer and nearer to that place toward which the Star guided them, they became very confident of arriving soon. They knew not exactly what lay at the end of the journey. But they felt destined to find what they had been seeking.

Suddenly, the camel stopped in his tracks and refused to go any farther. Hour after hour of coaxing, pushing and pulling was fruitless in getting him to move. A new day dawned, and stifling heat drained their last sources of energy. Finally, the glowing orb of the sun sank into the sand, and the firmament of stars spread over the dark blue dome above. The three wayfarers were totally defeated by the camel's stubbornness. They lay down and tried to sleep. What had gone wrong?

The night became cold, unfriendly, and they shivered in frustration. Who could help them? Certainly not the dumb animal. He was the cause of their problem. No, the camel was too stubborn to be of any further use. Yet, they could not continue, because none of the men could lead the way.

So, huddling together against the beast for warmth, they waited the inevitable end. Unable to sleep, all three became absorbed in personal reflections. Each experienced his life passing before him.

The blind man thought to himself, "How could we have failed?" He had offered his acute sense of hearing in the circle of trust and had diligently assisted the other two.

The deaf man reflected quietly upon the fact that in his trust he had given his keen power of sight to help the other two.

And the mute man, sunk in deep resignation, wondered how could his abilities have been without value? Hadn't he, through the trust, given his best gestures and firm touch of hand, so that they could reach their goal?

Adventures in Human Understanding

A sharp new breeze rose swiftly and started to howl. The noise became almost overpowering, and the journeymen began to feel as though they might perish at any moment. They formed once again the magic circle of trust, desperately clasping hands and turning their heads upwards. It was as though they were waiting for the Voice to guide them again, although they remembered that it had said, "I speak no more."

Then, above the howling wind, there came a wailing sound, eerie, unearthly. The trio stood up and, with all the trust, faith, and hope they could muster, they joined hands again. Perhaps the sound was that of the Voice relenting and once more rescuing them. They placed their arms about each other's shoulders in deep comradeship. Again the cry sounded out. It was a "bawwwww," like the bawling of a child in pain.

All at once, somehow, the journeymen knew from whence came that sound. The man with no eyes could almost see the anguish in the face of the camel. The deaf man could now almost hear the intensity of the camel's wail. And the mute man, with no speech, was almost able to speak a word of comfort to the poor, ungainly beast.

In a burst of enlightenment the men knew what the third and last rule of gold was to be. All three had, in criticizing each other's imperfections, failed to recognize the plight and need of that being, whom they now knew to be their best friend, the camel. They had all failed to think of "Charity."

All three of the journeymen now set fast to help a life other than themselves. Suddenly, the journey no longer seemed as important as they had once thought. It was far in the back of their minds whether they would ever find their way again or not. Here was a friend in need, and the three knew what they must do.

They all thought within themselves what it was that the Voice had once said, "I cannot give you that which you must find yourselves. You will do what you will do."

The three searchers for wisdom were just about to find it. Each one individually, yet acting together, set forth to do his job. Through their minds ran a common thread of understanding as each one thought, "I have acted in dependence of the other two for so long. I almost forgot my own abilities."

The deaf man, with his sensitive sight, noticed the camel's tongue swollen from thirst. The blind man, with the keen powers of his hearing, listened and heard the rustle of a small mound of hay nearby bracing itself against the wind. The man who was mute could see and hear that the poor beast was bawling and trembling from his sore and aching limbs, and he placed a hand of comfort on the camel.

So, it came to be. The deaf man, though he could not hear the camel's cry, lifted the water jug to the camel's mouth so as to quench his friend's thirst. The blind man groped until the hay was found and, touching the camel's head for guidance, fed his friend. And the mute man, through his touch, massaged the camel's sore limbs with olive oil.

After a period of rest for them all, they noticed again the heavenly star on the horizon, which was shining ever so brightly. The camel stood up and acknowledged its brilliance with one more "bawwwww," as if in a word of gratitude. He was, once again, as he had been, ready to lead the three men who were now his great friends. His strength was renewed, and he could now be the eyes, ears and touch for all of them. He would lead them to the end of their journey and to their reward. His own reward had been the kindness of their charity.

Following the camel's sure-fitted gait, the three travelers traversed the valley between the mountains to a place on a small hill just underneath the bright star. At this place, the camel folded his legs and came to rest on his knees. The three pilgrims also lowered themselves in respect as an amazing scene spread itself before them.

There below was a great gathering of countrymen and women, donkeys and other beasts of burden. They were all kneeling before a manger with a baby therein. And all was still.

Adventures in Human Understanding

Suddenly, from above the hill, there was a bright flash of lightning, and a deep rumble of thunder. They heard once more the commanding Voice.

"Oh, you three voyagers! You three blessed of men! I now make known my presence to you once more, even though you had not expected it. If you had, you might not have ever learnt the third and last of the rules of gold. It was something that each of you could discover only within your heart. You have discovered the value of your individual talents and abilities. The secret is "Charity." In helping someone other than yourselves in need, you have learnt that great things may happen. You have truly joined the brotherhood of mankind.

"You have also learnt how, through your deeds, you can enrich those who may be less fortunate in life. Now, without your new-found friend, the camel, who led you to this place, go forward together. All three of you can lead the way, side by side. For, Blind Man, you now have eyes that can see the beauties of this world. Deaf Man, the speech of others and the sounds of nature will come like music to your ears. Mute Man, you now have a voice with which to express your thoughts and share them with your fellowmen.

"Now look, you three! In the saddlebags on your friend, the camel, I have placed gifts for you to present to the one who lies in that manger. Rise now, and walk forward to present these gifts for you are now men of wisdom."

The Three Wise Men walked slowly, side by side, carrying their gifts down the hillside. All three were leading the way. Their friend, the camel, knelt quietly on the hilltop above.

As the three friends crept softly to the manger, they knelt and placed their gifts by the cradle. The bright yellow glow above the head of the child clearly revealed in utmost clarity a scene which they would never forget. Each of the Three Wise Men smiled to himself.

Yes, indeed, it had truly been A Golden Journey.

Thoughts of a Therapist: Analysis and Comment

John G. Watkins

The story's plot and characters were drawn from a well-known tale in biblical lore. However, this revision is more of an allegory. Its message, told in symbolic form, is the interdependence of us humans on each other and on other forms of life which share this earth. It is a tale of human interpersonal relationships.

Every individual has limitations, but the characters in this story each have a major disability, one which would keep them from attempting such a journey alone. They must first learn to trust one another.

In a crisis they seek support from a "Higher Power." The guidance that comes is not peculiar to any single religion: Christian, Jewish, Moslem or Buddhist. However, almost every person in the world believes there is order and meaning in the universe, which is controlled by some form of "Intelligence." There is room in this story for every contemporary faith—or even the polytheistic creeds of antiquity, Greek, Roman, Egyptian.

The understanding of three fundamental human values is required of the voyagers by this "Higher Power" before they can reach their goal: Faith, hope and charity. This "charity" must extend to all living creatures, not only themselves. By learning this lesson they are rewarded and reach their destination.

In the biblical version, the "Child" became the world's greatest teacher. Here, the child is meant to symbolize new life by which human disabilities are surmounted. The three men will finish their days in respected "wisdom."

This story is an appropriate termination point for our "Adventures in Human Understanding."

Other Titles from
Crown House Publishing
www.crownhouse.co.uk

Gestalt Therapy
The Attitude & Practice of an Atheoretical Experientialism
Claudio Naranjo, M.D.

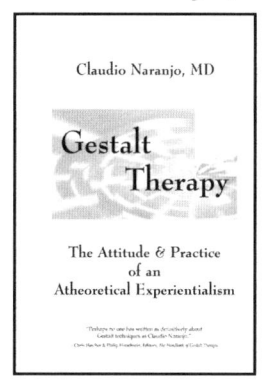

In this fascinating study, Naranjo has captured the flavour and distinctive character of the California-based school of Gestalt therapy, propagated by Perls in his last years as a teacher and exemplar of the approach he pioneered. Lively and highly readable, learned and insightful, this book is indispensable both for professionals and the lay-reader in demonstrating why Fritz Perls was truly the father of the now-flourishing human potential movement.

PAPER   320 PAGES   ISBN: 1899836543

"Perhaps no one has written as definitively about Gestalt techniques as Claudio Naranjo."—*Chris Hatcher and Philip Himelstein, Editors, The Handbook of Gestalt Therapy.*

Guided Imagery And Other Approaches To Healing
Rubin Battino, M.S.

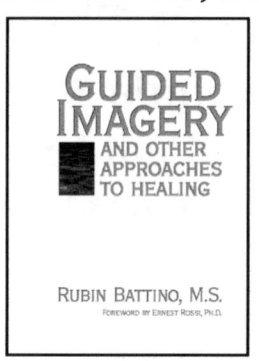

An essentially practical and accessible healing manual, **Guided Imagery** presents a breakdown of published guided imagery scripts, while investigating the language used in guided imagery, the skills required in rapport-building, and the most effective methods in inducing a state of relaxation. Pioneering new bonding and fusion healing methods, **Guided Imagery** also incorporates a useful section on preparing patients for surgery, and a chapter on Nutrition and Healing, by nutrition expert A. Ira Fritz, Ph.D., plus a chapter on Native American Healing Traditions, by Native American healer Helena Sheehan, Ph.D. Designed as a resource for health professionals, **Guided Imagery,** meticulously researched and authoritative, is essential reading for doctors, nurses, psychologists, counsellors and all those involved or interested in healing.

CLOTH 400 PAGES ISBN: 1899836446

"Well chosen, illuminating clinical examples abound, with eminently useful imagery suggestions for practitioner and patient."—*Belleruth Naparstek, L.I.S.W., author of Staying Well with Guided Imagery.*

Also available: two audiotape set of guided imagery scripts, 113 mins. ISBN: 1899836594

The Magic of Metaphor
77 Stories for
Teachers, Trainers & Thinkers
Nick Owen
with a foreword by Judith DeLozier

Presents a collection of powerful stories designed to engage, inspire and transform the listener and the reader, and a wealth of advice and information on the art of storytelling.

PAPER   320 PAGES   ISBN: 1899836705

"I think the book is a fine offering to the teaching and training world."—*Judith DeLozier, author, NLP developer.*

"A treasure trove of wisdom and fun! Stories for leaders to use on every occasion to enhance their effectiveness."
—*Richard D. Field, O.B.E., Industrialist, Leadership Coach and student.*

"The book appeals on diverse levels with insights and enlightening illustrations that will illuminate teaching and learning. Drawn from ancient oriental traditions, contemporary sources and the author's own repertoire—the experience is challenging, life-affirming and enriching."—*Mick Reid, Voluntary Service Overseas, London.*

The Power of Metaphor
Story Telling and Guided Journeys
for Teachers, Trainers & Therapists
Michael Berman & David Brown

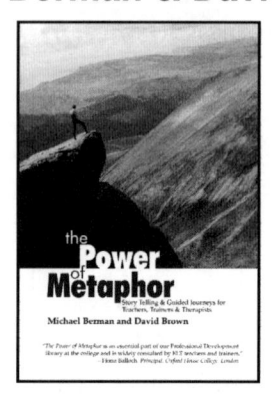

This unique book combines the power of metaphor and the dynamics of story telling. The metaphor is powerful because it parallels life; the story is dynamic because it captivates. When a metaphor is embedded in a story, the captivation of the listener activates the subconscious, and the metaphor is absorbed. Tracing techniques of story telling back to their original roots, it first promotes a deep understanding of the uses of metaphor, before presenting a series of enjoyable and thought-provoking stories. Each story takes the form of a guided journey that leads the listener along an imaginative path. Each forms a script for an inspiring story session that will enhance the learning of its listeners. Packed with original stories and visualisations, **The Power of Metaphor** is an invaluable resource for teachers, trainers and therapists. If you are looking for new approaches to group work, or if you are interested in the art of story telling, this book will prove an illuminating and stimulating read.

PAPER   216 PAGES   ISBN: 1899836438

"**The Power of Metaphor** is an essential part of our Professional Development library at the college and is widely consulted by ELT teachers and trainers."—*Fiona Balloch, Principal, Oxford House College, London.*

The Structure of Personality
Modelling "Personality" Using NLP and Neuro-Semantics
L. Michael Hall, Ph.D., Bob G. Bodenhamer, D.Min., Richard Bolstad & Margot Hamblett

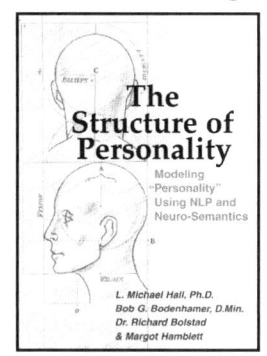

The Structure of Personality identifies the process of producing a personality, and presents strategies that will reprogram personality. Coaching the reader in a number of effective and specially adapted NLP techniques, it includes tools such as The R.E.S.O.L.V.E. model and the Personal Strengths model, making it an essential reference for counsellors, therapists and NLP practitioners.

CLOTH   496 PAGES   ISBN: 1899836675

"A bold and courageous step with exciting possibilities. The authors have dismantled the diagnostic nomenclature offering new perspectives for treatment while postulating that personality is not static; not a thing, but an ongoing, evolving process and, if dysfunctional, can be restructured. The book should prove to be a milestone in our pursuit for sanity."—*Rie Anderson, M.A., L.M.H.C., N.B.C.D.C.H., Clinical Psychotherapist.*

"*The Structure of Personality* is a major step in creating a cognitive map using Neuro-Semantics and Neuro-Linguistic Programming to understand the relationship between a person's thinking and his or her personality development."
—*Jim Walsh, M.A., Licensed Mental Health Counselor, Certified School Psychologist, Certified Neuro-Semantics and Neuro-Linguistics Trainer.*

USA & Canada *orders to:*

LPC Group
22 Broad Street, Suite 34, Milford, CT 06460
Tel: 800-626-4330, Fax: 800-334-3892
www.lpcgroup.com

UK & Rest of World *orders to:*

The Anglo American Book Company Ltd.
Crown Buildings, Bancyfelin, Carmarthen, Wales SA33 5ND
Tel: +44 (0)1267 211880/211886, Fax: +44 (0)1267 211882
E-mail: books@anglo-american.co.uk
www.anglo-american.co.uk

Australasia *orders to:*

Footprint Books Pty Ltd
101 McCarrs Creek Road, PO Box 418, Church Point
Sydney NSW 2105, Australia
Tel: +61 2 9997 3973, Fax: +61 2 9997 3185
E-mail: footprintbooks@ozmail.com.au